Natural & Organic Healing

Your Ultimate Guide to Health & Wellness
2019

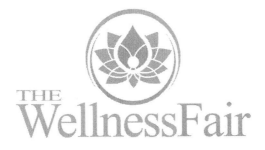

www.TheWellnessFair.org

organized by: Lucas J. Robak

Co-Authors From Wisconsin & Beyond

Copyright © 2019 Authored by Lucas J. Robak
Published by The Wellness Fair
All rights reserved.

This publication is designed to provide competent and reliable information regarding the subject matter covered. However, it is sold with the understanding that the author, co-authors, and publisher are not engaged in rendering medical, health, or other professional advice. If medical or other expert assistance is required, the services of a professional should be sought. The author, co-authors, and publisher specifically disclaim any liability that is incurred from the use or application of the contents in this book. Think for yourself and chose your own actions!

Also available at Amazon.com and www.TheWellnessFair.org to purchase paperback.

Downloadable pdf is available on our co-authors websites.

ASIN: 1687046506
ISBN: 9781687046505

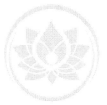

Contributing Wellpreneurs

Leslie Zapf Desrosiers
Lucas J. Robak
Sheila Pryce Brooks
Misa Tsuyoshi
Kim Farmer
Dr. Karen Valentin
Marquita h Catallo-Madruga
Luanne Nelson
Alexis Dowd
Reina Rose
Jory Pradjinski
Heather Hirschman
Archana Amlapure
Kathleen Mulligan
Dr. Karen Stillman
Ursula Wood
Patti Beres
Aprilani McIlwraith
Amy Carter
Kelli Hirt
Vivianne Romang
Kelly Brickel
Vivian Jalique

*"So many people spend their health gaining wealth,
and the have to spend their wealth to regain their health."*
~ A.J. Reb Materi ~

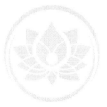

About The Wellness Fair

The Wellness Fair unites accredited wellness professionals with those who desire complete well-being. Our community naturally integrates the health of the whole body; physical, mental, emotional, and spiritual.

Online Wellness

Whether it's by attending our local trade fairs and speaking events or going online to consume the wisdom our community shares, you're bound to find that one golden nugget you need to improve your overall wellness.

There are various ways you can learn from our International qualified wellness professionals. You already started by picking up this book. Every November 1st, we release that years anthology book on Amazon. Mark your calendars because only in the month of November are all the volumes discounted for holiday gifts.

By going to our website, you'll also gather a great deal of information through our guest blog, *Thriving Naturally*. Every quarter we also release a new issue of our digital magazine, *Pathways 2 Wellness*. Finally, if you're really not the reading type, you're able to learn from practitioners from around the world on our podcast, *Healthy Conversations*.

Local Events

Attendees now have the ability to join our community to connect with service providers, learn a variety of health tips, and have their voice heard whenever it's convenient for them.

Our annual trade fairs consist of educational classes, workshops, and presentations to empower you to live a healthier lifestyle. To maintain the highest quality for you, all our presenters are chosen one month before the fair during our speakers conference called, *The Speakers Jam.*

Thousands of attendees are able to connect with hundreds of wellness practitioners all year. Visit our website and mark your calendars.

Getting Active

There are many ways you can get involved with our community:

1. Attend events as a wellness enthusiast
2. Consume our wisdom sharing materials
3. Be a vendor at a local trade fair nearest you
4. Once a vendor, you're able to be a speaker
5. Become a co-author in the next volume of this book series
6. Contribute to our guest blog
7. Contribute to our quarterly magazine
8. Be a guest on our podcast
9. Volunteer
10. Sponsor
11. Acquire a license to host events in your area

By partnering with us, you can leverage our community for an entire career; we'll train you how.

Does this seem like something you would be interested in?

Go to www.TheWellnessFair.org and sign up today.

Thank you!

Dedication

This book is dedicated to all those seeking a natural and healthy lifestyle. We hope you find that one golden nugget to improve your spiritual, mental, emotional, physical, or business well-being.

Table of Contents

Dr. Leslie Desrosiers, DPT, OCS, CSCS

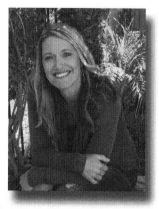

Dr. Leslie is a Doctor of Physical Therapy, Orthopedic Specialist, and sports injury prevention expert.

She owns *Elite Concepts Physical Therapy and Performance*, a concierge private practice, where she helps active people live the lives of their dreams by resolving painful conditions, improving mobility, and getting them back to the activities they want to do.

She has extensive experience with all ages and abilities, including youth to professional athletes.

Dr. Leslie developed *ACL Strong*, an online program helping athletes protect their knees and prevent injuries so they can thrive in sports for life.

Outside of providing specialized one-on-one care, consulting on injury prevention, and writing for various publications, Dr. Leslie enjoys spending time with her family and living the San Diego lifestyle.

*"Physical strength is the most important thing in life.
This is true whether we want it to be or not."*
~ Mark Rippetoe ~

San Diego, California, USA

Website: www. aclstrong.com
Website: www.eliteconceptspt.com

Social Media:
- www.facebook.com/ACLSTRONG
- www.facebook.com/EliteConceptsPT
- www.linkedin.com/in/lesliedesrosiers

Natural & Organic Healing

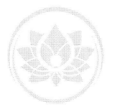

Foreword

Prehab over Rehab
How Prevention Can Help You Reach Your Dreams

We all want to be free to live the lives of our dreams!

We want to do the activities we love without anything getting in our way.

Whether your goal is to compete in a high-level sport, travel and explore the world, or simply play on the floor with your grandchildren, we all want to do *something*.

Let's be honest, we don't have patience for hurdles. We get frustrated with detours and angry or discouraged with road-blocks.

What if I told you there was a simple solution to enhance the likelihood of your dreams becoming reality?

It's something so straight-forward that most people aren't doing it.

Prevention

The problem is, when it comes to prevention, most people think they're "too busy", "too tired", or they "don't need it."

You've heard the old saying, "If it isn't broke, don't fix it", right? When it comes to your health and wellness, it's actually quite wrong.

Instead, we should put a higher priority on preventative maintenance to keep our bodies functioning and performing at optimal potential.

Change the oil. Rotate your tires. Don't let your car sit in the garage for years without starting the engine. Have you heard those tips before?

You tune-up your car so it doesn't break-down...you go to the dentist to prevent cavities...you take your children for well-checks even when they aren't sick...Why wouldn't you protect your own body from injury, illness, or aging, before it's too late?

As a Doctor of Physical Therapy and sports injury prevention expert; I help active people prevent or quickly recover from injury so they can thrive in their sports and in life without annoying setbacks. I help them manage their bodies, keep their joints healthy, and perform their best.

I am passionate about helping athletes prevent injuries so they are capable of reaching their dreams and competing at a higher level, because getting hurt leads to wasting time on the sidelines instead of excelling in their sport. They lose opportunities to advance, win championships, or earn scholarships.

Research has proven extensively that "injury prevention training" reduces injuries and enhances performance. Period.

Athletes are beginning to recognize that "prehab is much easier than rehab," meaning you can spend a little time to prevent an injury, rather than waste a lot of time rehabilitating from one.

While you may not be chasing a college scholarship, you have your own goals for living your best life. Whatever your dreams are, there are strategies to help you get there by improving your health and wellness, and preventing decline.

There is something for everyone when it comes to strategies to improve your health and wellness, naturally!

What you need to watch out for, however, is *overwhelm*. Sometimes having so much information at our disposal can become overwhelming, confusing, and can stop us from making any decision at all.

The reality is, there is no "one-size-fits-all" approach to health and wellness. We are all unique individuals with different goals.

The key to finding the best health and wellness plan for you, is by trying different strategies that fit your lifestyle.

Rather than relying on one approach to fix all of your problems, wellness is about overlay of multiple strategies that aim to improve your health from different perspectives. Consider applying a few different strategies to enhance your overall health, fitness, and well-being. Make sure your strategies fit your life so you make wellness a long-term lifestyle change, not a temporary binge diet that's impossible to sustain.

When I first learned about Lucas Robak's interest in *Natural & Organic Healing*, I saw how his commitment to life-long learning and passion for holistic health changed his life. He is a genuine example of someone who took charge of his life through health and wellness; and he is dedicated to helping others do the same. He understands that finding solutions for pain, illness, and aging can be confusing, exhausting, and intimidating.

Through his development of *The Wellness Fair*, authoring several books, organizing events, and leading support groups, Lucas has helped thousands of people find inspiration, take charge of their health, and achieve the active lifestyles of their dreams.

Natural & Organic Healing makes it easy for anyone to discover and learn more about *Natural & Organic Healing* remedies. From meditation to nutrition, from technology to mindset, and from hope to action, Lucas cuts through the clutter and brings together niche experts from around the world to provide clarity for achieving your health, fitness, and lifestyle goals.

If you want to live the life of your dreams, and not let injuries, illness, or aging get in your way, now is the time to switch to a proactive mindset – choose prehab over rehab, prevention over rehabilitation, and a variety of natural health and wellness strategies that fit your lifestyle.

This book will transform you from feeling overwhelmed, exhausted, and defeated by health issues, to feeling confident and empowered to live a life of *Natural & Organic Healing*.

Here's to you achieving the future of your dreams.

Enjoy!

Lucas J. Robak

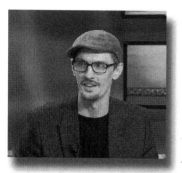

As a former pilot, wine maker, and teacher, Lucas J. Robak is a #1 bestselling author and a contributor to numerous publications like *Addicted 2 Success*, *Good Men Project*, and *Thrive Global*.

After publishing 75 people around the world for fun, he saw a need and is now considered to be the Entrepreneurs Publisher with *Authorpreneur Academy*.

A diagnosis of multiple sclerosis (MS) motivated Lucas to become a leader of *The Wellness Fair* by connecting qualified wellness professionals to those who desire a natural and healthy lifestyle.

This book series is a way for him to fulfill his purpose, "to help people become aware of their bodies natural ability to heal itself." Enjoy!

"You will continue to suffer if you have an emotional reaction to everything that is said to you. True power is sitting back and observing things with logic. True power is restraint. If words control you that means everyone else can control you. Breathe and allow things to pass."
~ Cindy Flores ~

Milwaukee, Wisconsin, USA

Website: www.LucasRobak.com

Social Media:
- www.linkedin.com/in/LucasJRobak/
- www.facebook.com/LucasJRobak
- www.instagram.com/LucasJRobak

Enjoy growing as a person? Me too! Check out this list of my Top 150 Recommended Books (no email required) www.LucasRobak.com/150books

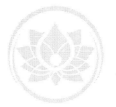

Introduction

"You can't connect the dots looking forward; you can only connect them looking backwards. So you have to trust that the dots will somehow connect in your future. You have to trust in something - your gut, destiny, life, karma, whatever. This approach has never let me down, and it has made all the difference in my life."
~ Steve Jobs ~

Imagine this! You're sitting alone in a hospital bed because you chose not to tell anyone you're checking yourself into one of their weekend suites.

What brought you to the Emergency Room that evening is one side of your body decided to stop working for a couple weeks; and it now hurts like hell.

Everyday you're exhausted the moment you wake up. Thinking is now a chore. Walking a straight line is near impossible, even using a walker is finally out of the question. Holding something in your hands, well, forget about that one, your left hand doesn't work anymore. Want to read something? Have someone read it to you instead because of how blurred your vision is. Make sure you clear your calendar when it's time to go to the bathroom, it could take an hour to start going and even longer to stop. Your short term memory is on strike, but only when it wants to be. To make sure life is even more interesting by creating embarrassing moments, remembering the names and faces of those you already know becomes questionable.

This was my life before a team of neurologists in the stroke unit at Froedtert Hospital in Milwaukee, WI handed me my life's purpose on a silver platter.

Hi! I'm Lucas J. Robak, the organizer of *The Wellness Fair* and the organizing author of this book series, *Natural & Organic Healing*.

I was gifted with the diagnosis of multiple sclerosis (MS) on May 30, 2014.

What is MS? I don't care what it is nor do I care about what it could possibly, might potentially do to me at some unforeseen point in the future. That knowledge is useless and pointless to me. I'm not a doctor, have never played one on T.V., and I didn't stay at a Holiday Inn Express last night. It's not my job to know anything about MS.

The only thing that matters is what's 100% in my control. How do I successfully live with one of the most debilitating neurological disorders known to mankind? The answer, this book and everything else I'm doing with my life!

The only challenge I've come across with developing this mentality is there are more than enough people out there who consistently force information on me which was never asked for. It's as if people purposefully want me to choose to become a hypochondriac so they can feel even worse for me. Don't make yourself out to be the victim due to my thinking. I'm not a victim of MS until I consciously choose to make that decision for myself.

Years leading up to that glorious moment at Froedtert, I was digging deep within myself to discover my purpose in life after attempting suicide in college. From experience, I knew it wasn't doing what society told me to do. Already did all that and it's not for me, hence the suicide attempt.

The beautiful Earl Nightingale tells me on a daily basis through his audio-book, *The Strangest Secret*, "The opposite of courage in our society is not cowardice... it is conformity." I spent a huge chunk of my life living like a conformed coward and it almost killed me.

Every now and then Art Williams pops in my life to say 'hi' through his 1987 speech, *Just Do It*. He loves reminding me, "... the only way not to be controversial is to be average and ordinary. Just call me anything but average and ordinary."

"If I want to be free, I've gotta be me. Not the me I think you think I should be. Not the me I think my wife thinks I should I be. Not the me I think my kids think I should be. But if I want to be free, I've gotta be. So I'd better know who me is."
~ Bill Gove ~

I personally believe that conformity is a mental illness. The reason being is because when you do what your told, think what you're told to think, and act the way society demands you to act, you're not you - you're doing what the people in power dictate down to you instead; you're controlled by others.

The person who you're truly meant to be is dying inside because you want society to look upon as "one of us." Well, thankfully, I'm not you, I'm me!

And if I wanna be free, I've gotta be me!

Once I started down the path of "being me," that's when everything started to come together … and fall apart.

What fell apart were most of my prior relationships, we were no longer thinking and functioning on the same frequency. We either naturally drifted away from each other, or I purposefully burnt the bridge to end that negative part of my life.

What came together, was me! Through books, videos, seminars, conferences, writing with a pen on paper, and a lot of status quo resistance, I deliberately transformed my life into what I consciously mapped out.

Before continuing, I'd like to make clear that I'm not saying suicide or chronic illnesses are a positive thing, they're not. What I've intentionally reprogrammed myself to do is to seek out the positives buried within the negatives; make this simple decision and you can easily do it too.

If I never attempted suicide, I never would have started down the path of personal development. I never would have came to realize first-hand how powerful we all are. Without medication, and without therapy, I thought myself out of depression and into the life you're seeing today. I chose to do it this way because I figured if one can think themselves into suicide, just imagine the possibilities of what you can think yourself into on the positive end of the spectrum.

Now onto my glorious MS, the real reason you have this book in your hands.

For over a decade I trained myself to ignore my body because I equated it to be like my car, if you keep driving, that "clunk" will fix itself … and it does every time. In 2014 I came to realize that when my body "fixed itself," that was just an active lesion in my brain or spine dying off.

I'm sure you're somewhat the same too. Every time your body tries to tell you something, do you actually listen and do something about it or just keep going about your life like I did?

Metaphorically speaking, my body was beating the hell out of me and I took like a champ - I thought everyone experienced this. I didn't want to be one of those people who go to the ER just because I blew my nose. By the way, due to MS, I'm always the healthiest person in every room because my immune system is stronger than it should be. What does "blowing your nose" even mean? Can't remember the last time that happened to me. Jealous of my MS yet?

While sitting in the hospital bed for three days, once I was done working, I found time to start researching MS. After reading the first sentence in my first search I instantly learned to stop looking up MS. Instead, I started researching how to successfully live with a chronic illness.

Guess what I found? Exactly what we all should be doing in the first place!

Natural, organic, Eastern medicine ... preventative care! There's no need to swallow a bunch of pills if you actually take care of yourself, right?

Personally, I believe the only reason this isn't mainstream yet is because there isn't billions of dollars to be made and no patents can be filed. The pharmaceutical companies, lobbyists, politicians, FDA officials, hospitals, and nonprofits stand to lose hundreds of billions of dollars every year once the world wakes up to natural health and their bodies innate ability to heal itself without doing hardcore drugs. Western medicine would cease to exist outside the ER and diagnostics.

This is my goal, my purpose in life, my obligation to the world!

Without going to the Lobbyist store and making an expensive purchase to legally own the decisions of a few politicians and numerous FDA officials, we can achieve this goal of perfect health by simply gaining the knowledge provided within this book series.

My obligation in life: "to help the world become aware of their bodies natural ability to heal itself." And I'm not going to be the one delivering the message, nor the one working one-on-one with people; let's leave that to the professionals in this book series.

> "The best way to predict the future is to create it."
> ~ Abraham Lincoln ~

To achieve my purpose in life, I'm the back seat driver. Instead of me striving to be the next big thing in the wellness world; I work with wellpreneurs to help them effectively reach more people.

Even though I have my master practitioner certification in Neuro-Linguistic Programming (NLP), master hypnotherapist certification, and Reiki Level II certification; instead of me working with you directly pertaining to your health goals, I'm now working with wellness professionals for them to gain more visibility and credibility in the marketplace so you can find them easier.

Do you like what you've read from a particular co-author?

Reach out and hire them - they'd do a far better job with you than I ever could! I'm simply just a community organizer and entrepreneur publisher. The co-authors are the ones who'll be there to change your life, it's no longer me.

- Thankfully, I attempted suicide.
- Thankfully, I developed and become aware of MS.
- Thankfully, I chose to create the mentality I did to seek the positives when society wants you to choose victimhood instead.

Because of all this, *The Wellness Fair* exists. Because of all this, you're reading a wonderful book filled with imperative information, that once converted to knowledge through implementation, could revolutionize your entire well-being.

Enjoy this book, read the other books within the *Natural & Organic Healing* series, connect with all the contributing authors, and at some point, I'll be seeing you at our next wellness event!

With love and appreciation,

Lucas J. Robak

Community Organizer
www.TheWellnessFair.org/Lucas

Sheila Pryce Brooks

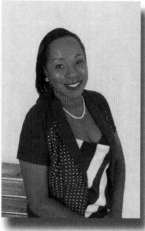

After secretly living with sleep paralysis for over 30 years, Sheila decided to break her silence about her struggle by writing a self-help book for persons who experience sleep paralysis, or those seeking more information.

The book is called: *Beyond the Nightmare: How to Transcend Sleep Paralysis and Awaken Your Spiritual Gifts.*

In this book she shares the methods used to transform her life.

Sleep paralysis has brought about a deeply personal and spiritual transformation.

Sheila has continually unfolding spiritual and psychic abilities, and as the Internet's leading voice working with the spiritual side of sleep paralysis, she not only provides support and alternative options to those suffering from sleep paralysis, but Sheila also expands the current thinking.

*"I learned that courage was not the absence of fear, but the triumph over it.
The brave man is not he who does not feel afraid,
but he who conquers that fear."
~ Nelson Mandela ~*

Junction P.O., St. Elizabeth, Jamaica

Website: www.sheilaprycebrooks.com

Social Media:
- www.facebook.com/sheilaprycebrooks/
- www.linkedin.com/in/sheila-pryce-brooks-9a810128/
- www.instagram.com/sheilaprycebrooks/

Don't be a victim to sleep paralysis. Book a free consultation now.

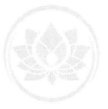

Beyond the Nightmare

My eyes open sharply as if startled awake. My mind struggles to catch up, lagging behind, as my eyes see dimmed darkness all around and my skin feels the coolness of the air. Still trying to make sense of the scene, my eyes search for markers, anything that will help me identify where I am.

And then my mind catches up .... I realise I'm still asleep. But how can that be? As the thought comes to me, so too does the panic. If I am still asleep then where am I?

The panic increases as unanswered questions aid my confusion, and the panic changes to fear as I attempt to move; only to find that my arms, legs, and torso are rigid, paralysed. Unable to move, terror sets in where there once was fear.

As my eyes dart from side to side the terror increases as I sense an audience. But not a human audience. They are dark, hunched, and the eyes. I can see the eyes in the darkness.

A foreboding comes over me. Instinctively I know I have to leave this place, and quickly. Something evil is here and I am the focus of its attention. As I try to move again, I feel a weight pressing down against my chest. Sheer horror overtakes me as I look upon a great beast astride me.

I am a witness to my own nightmare.
That is sleep paralysis!

It is estimated that 4 out of every 10 people globally have sleep paralysis episodes with little or no help in sight. There seems to be no criteria to make one person more likely than another to experience it and cases have been identified all over the world with males and females equally affected.

There are some studies which state over half the global population will experience an episode of sleep paralysis. The episodes do not occur singularly, but are in fact, repetitive. They take place sporadically and there is no pattern or factor to determine their frequency. If they take place once, they have or will take place again.

Considering the number of persons experiencing this phenomenon, it is poorly understood, and millions of people are in search of answers and a 'cure' to stop the attacks.

For those who experience sleep paralysis, a definition is not necessary. In fact, defining it creates unwanted anxiety, as memories and feelings are relived with the terror in which they were created.

To the experienced, definitions cement the fact that 'it' actually happened. That 'it' was not a hallucination and the quandary creates the realisation that perhaps, unworldly, spiritual and ghoulish entities exist, which cannot be controlled, let alone defined.

When we review the history of sleep paralysis, we find it has been known about for hundreds of years with its formal written recognition in The American Academy of Sleep Medicine's first publication in 1979 This is where it was classified as a 'sleep and arousal' disorder.

Going back even further, sleep paralysis was highlighted in an oil painting by Henry Fuseli in 1781, called The Nightmare where he depicts a demonic incubus sitting on a sleeping woman's chest; her arms and head thrown below her, whilst a black horse looks on. This scene is commonly witnessed by the sleep paralysis sufferer.

According to sleep experts, the phenomena consist of some or all of the following whilst sleeping:

- The sleeper senses an evil presence in the room, which is threatening and intimidating;
- The sleeper feels something pressing down on their chest or abdomen;
- The sleeper is unable to move a muscle or utter a sound;
- The sleeper feels that they are being choked or strangled;
- The sleeper feels themselves outside of their body and can float or fly. They can also see themselves from above.

To anyone who has not experienced sleep paralysis, this definition of something that actually takes place may sound utterly ridiculous, impossible, and incomprehensible. The normal response is: 'he/she must have been dreaming,' or 'they're going through a stressful time which triggered a nightmare.' The most ironic response is 'you just need a good nights' sleep!'

But, how is it explained when these 'nightmares' happen over and over again, night after night? When there's no storyline or plot in the dream, no characters apart from the dreamer and the intruder/s? When there are no 'stressful situations' or personal problems? When the individual is perfectly healthy and everything else in their life is going well?

The sleep paralysis experiencer normally keeps their episodes to themselves. They are apprehensive to discuss it for several reasons; fear of being misunderstood, fear of appearing 'strange or weird' and even fear of being likened to having an infectious disease that must be kept secret. Hoping that if no one finds out, they can continue to be 'normal'. Privately they search for help. Google search after Google, bookstore after bookstore, hoping to find what isn't there.

The sufferer will avoid doctors with their 'spooky illness' unless it becomes absolutely unbearable and doctors who are determined to avoid spiritual mysticism, are focused on conventional methods, many not knowing what to do about it and many never having heard of it before, as a medical condition, that is.

The life of someone who experiences sleep paralysis is plagued with constant tiredness and fatigue due to not only lack of sleep, but also disturbed sleep. It's also important to note there are no determinants of regularity, they can take place weekly, bi-monthly or yearly. Fear of sleeping, fear of the dark, and fear of the night time are common. The impact of sleep paralysis on the everyday person is hard. With little to nil support and no treatments nearby the phenomena continues as it has done for over 2,000 years.

As a chronic suffer of sleep paralysis for over 30 years, the frightening visitations have now subsided, replaced by a spiritual awakening, triggered by the psychic engagement. I have metamorphosed with clarity, enlightenment and understanding of the experience which has renewed my outlook, not only on the sleep paralysis episode, but on the spiritual world we are an intrinsic part of.

The sleep paralysis experience is hinged with the human spirit and Universal intervention. The nature of us being 'human spiritual beings' has been well documented, with many scientific and spiritual teachers from different approaches each emphasising the same thing; that we are spiritual in the first instance, with the human physical body providing a shell for the spiritual energy which is the overriding part of our makeup.

This spiritual energy is the underpinning perspective when explaining the 'hows' and 'whys' of sleep paralysis. This spiritual energy and its unique frequency vary from person to person, to the extent that no two people are alike.

The determinants of your energetic frequency are many and you have the ability to increase or decrease it. Generally, the lower frequencies represent negative emotions and feelings such as; depression, sadness, pessimism, negative thoughts etc. The higher frequencies represent; positive thoughts, happiness, joy, and love.

When it comes to spiritual energy, you also need to factor in the energies which are ever present and interacting with each of us constantly. This energy moves, fluctuates, and mixes with us unceasingly, intertwining with your spiritual energy, continually calling your attention in the form of your intuition, signs, increased perception or synchronicities.

These broader external energies (we will call them source energy for now) exists at an extremely high frequency, which is why it is often difficult for us to clearly interact and hear the calling being offered. As for most of us, our spiritual energy operates at a lower frequency to that of the source energy.

Whilst we sleep, our spiritual energy interacts free of resistance with the source energy and engages the broader spiritual, energetic, world.

For some of us the experience is seamless, and we awaken none the wiser with whispers of events that took place. But there are some of us, those who experience sleep paralysis, who have a far more intense experience, the source of spiritual energy attempts to engage us at a higher energetic frequency than we are ready for.

As the sleep paralysis experiencer sleeps, with relatively clear resistance, the broader source energies attempt to engage them – to capture their attention. The energy frequency being emitted at that time is too low to comprehend and make sense of during the sleep state. The sleeper enters into a state of shock, which is compounded by the body's physiological response of paralysis and they awaken in the spiritual or sleep realm unable to comprehend what has taken place.

The shock and panic of the experience throws the sleeper into a state of fear and panic which can be likened to being thrown into a cold bath whilst asleep. Whilst in shock, the mind creates a framework for the fear, which is partly physiological - the paralysis, and entities are seen as the mind tries to make sense of the experience. The sleeper unwittingly rejects the energy, interpreting it negatively, as they force themselves awake saying: "What the hell just happened?".

Fortunately, there are practices that can reduce sleep paralysis and unlock the spiritual gifts. As you complete these practices, your sleep paralysis will subside as 'other' more positive spiritual experiences will take place, both during the wake and sleep state. You begin to see miracles. Literally!

Misa Tsuyoshi

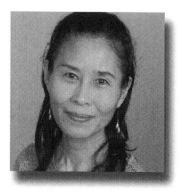

Misa has been a student of internationally recognized Qigong Grand Master, Chunyi Lin, and Spring Forest Qigong after her recovery from cancer in 2013.

She loves to share Qigong which has changed her lifestyle, perceptions, and relationships.

She is a certified Spring Forest Qigong Instructor / Trainer / Healer, a Certified Original Tai Chi Fundamentals® Program Instructor, Certified Tai Chi Fundamentals® Adapted Program Basic Moves and Short Form Instructor, a certified AFAA Personal Trainer, and a meditation facilitator.

She was recognized by Spring Forest Qigong as "Certified Qigong Trainer of The Year" (2018), and "Teacher of The Year" (2019).

"Energy cannot be created or destroyed,
it can only be changed from one form to another."
~ Albert Einstein ~

Brookfield, Wisconsin, USA

Website: www.simplewellnessfacilitator.com/

Social Media:
- www.facebook.com/pg/SimpleWellnessFacilitator/
- www.linkedin.com/in/misa-t-653b46166/

One stop modality for your healing and wellness-from the energy level and up
simplewellnessfacilitator@gmail.com

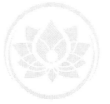

8 Reasons to Try
Spring Forest Qigong for Healing

In Japan, we say (on-co-chi-shin) when we learn something new by visiting something old.

As I study Spring Forest Qigong (SFQ), created by Grand Master Chunyi Lin, I am amazed to experience how this Qigong, which can be explained to Western people as a "Thousands year old Quantum Healing", is easy to learn and incorporate into my daily life. It has helped me to connect with the universal wisdom. It has been continuing to help me heal, prevent illnesses, help others, and guide me to be a better human.

In 2012 I started practicing SFQ while I was recovering from a cancer removal surgery. I have been cancer-free since then. I did not need to go through a recommended therapy and the doctor was very impressed. (Note: I am not suggesting you do SFQ instead of recommended therapy/medication/procedure by your doctor. This is my personal story).

Since then, I have learned more with Master Lin. I became a Certified Instructor/Trainer/Healer and have seen my lifestyle/perception change. I also started to attract more opportunities that are aligned with my life purpose as a healer and a teacher. I am feeling guided and blessed.

There are Thousands of Qigong. Why SFQ?

1. Most ancient Qigong are complicated and take a long time to learn. I heard students saying "the Qigong master practices four hours a day for decades. Not for me." Not so with SFQ.

2. Their techniques were kept secret—it was the way Asian traditions were passed on (especially martial arts and healing arts like Qigong). Only a selected few were allowed to learn the core principles/techniques of the modality.

As an outsider, you might learn a movement but may not know what the benefits really are other than "balancing energy".

3. Most Qigong have only movements. Throughout history, many meditations have been treated as closely guarded secrets.

Master Lin broke from ancient traditions and created SFQ because he strongly believes that "Qigong is such a powerful tool for healing, the whole world needs to know about it and benefit from it."

How SFQ stands out?

Master Lin found out through his own sufferings and healing journey that "the simplest things are the most powerful" and received the message/vision: 'A healer in every home. The world without pain and suffering."

He decided to create a simplified Qigong and share what he had learned in the past decades. SFQ was born. I was fortunate to learn the wealth of wisdom Master Lin has been selflessly sharing, and decided to share it by teaching classes/seminars as a certified SFQ instructor/healer not only because I have tremendously benefited from it but:

- Helps everyone to be his/her own wellness and healing facilitator by waking up the inner natural ability to heal. We can speed up recovery from a surgery or medical procedure. SFQ provides self-care techniques, therefore, we can take control of our own maintenance.

- Helps us to exercise loving others unconditionally, forgiving, and being kind to ourselves and others ... with compassion. We go deeper into our soul.

- SFQ is not intended to replace any medical procedure, therapy, medicines. It complements what we are already doing.

- It is not related to any religion and works well with any religion/belief.

- It offers tools such as active exercises (moving meditation), guided meditation, breathing techniques, as well as, an abundance of simple and easy self-care techniques; such as, massaging or cupping specific body parts for a specific condition. It works on the root cause of a condition.

- Research by medical doctors show a positive outcome: that SFQ is especially effective in pain/stress reduction. We all know stress is the major cause of illnesses. SFQ helps us to reduce stress before a physical symptom manifests.

- Many doctors have also witnessed "miracle healing stories" they could not explain.

- Meditations are to relax our body and mind. SFQ Meditation works deeper at a cellular level and facilitates healing. Why so? SFQ uses visualizations and messages. It is designed to open our hearts and activate our Unconditional Love Energy, which is the most powerful healing energy. It also connects us with the Universal/Divine/Your God's Unconditional Love, which makes our healing more powerful. It helps our consciousness to come forward and connect us with the Universal consciousness—we will be guided.

- SFQ is the first Qigong form in history that has successfully integrated the five elements with emotions. This integration immediately brings you to the highest level to balance the body, because emotions direct the energy flow of the body.

- Spring Forest Qigong is also able to explain why certain principles work. Master Lin developed the Seven Dimensions © to help explain advanced concepts of Spring Forest Qigong.

Eight Reasons to Try SFQ

1. SFQ does not take time. Practicing 30 minutes to one hour a day would be ideal. However, five minutes of moving meditation can do wonders when you are stressed or in pain.

2. Simplified for modern people. No equipment or special space required. Not even a mat. Just relax and move your hands or follow the meditation CD to balance energy and facilitate healing.

3. It works on the root cause, not the symptom—symptoms will go away completely when you work on the root cause and balance energy. You will learn how to find the root cause and how to work on it. As you continue to practice, you can balance the energy before any imbalance can manifest physically. SFQ can prevent illnesses.

4. It gives you the tools you can incorporate into your daily life.

5. You can facilitate your healing and other's healing. In advanced SFQ classes, you will learn in-person healing and long-distance healing.

6. No need for other modalities—it is complete with daily exercises (moving meditation), healing technique and meditation as well as lifestyle suggestions.

7. It uses something everyone has— "I want to stay well/live long/be healed". Anyone can do it. SFQ is a "Message Healing" "Information Healing". Your intention will help you to create messages which transform certain energy forms such as pains/illnesses/negative emotions/trauma back to normal. SFQ works the energy. Energy does not judge and flows where the mind goes. Even if you do not believe it, it still works. If you believe it, the healing will be more powerful.

8. It wakes up your forgotten love. You do not need to seek love from others. You will recognize you are the love. You will become a "love radiator".

Sample SFQ Self-Care and Healing Techniques

Yin-Yang Water:
Taoist medicine water balances energy and helps the digestive system. Pour boiling water and room temperature water (same amount) in a cup. Drink while it is warm. You can add a small amount of pure honey (considered to be a medicine).

Energy Breathing:
Slow down your breaths. Inhale and let the lungs expand. Exhale and try to empty the lungs while relaxing the lower abdomen. As you inhale, visualize beautiful lights or supporting energy coming through every part of the body, collecting in your Lower Dantian (vitality energy center deep in behind the navel). Exhale, visualize everything (negative emotion/experience/ pain / sickness) is changing into smoke and going out of the body.

Cupping the Tailbone and Kidneys with Loose Fists:
By cupping (or rubbing with the palms), you can strengthen your vitality. If you are sitting all day long, it would be helpful to do this every so often, ideally once every 30 minutes. Tip forward from the hips (to prevent the vibration from going into the brain directly), cup gently around the tailbone area, which is considered as a gateway to the vitality energy. After 2-5 minutes, cup gently around the kidneys. The kidney energy channel governs our vitality energy, and cupping this area helps strengthen our vitality.

Above are just the only three branches taken from the big forest.

*""--in Emptiness, Body, Feelings, Perceptions, Mental Formations
and Consciousness are not separate self-entities."*
~ Quan Yin Heart Sutra ~
(translated by Thich Nhat Hanh)

Kim Farmer

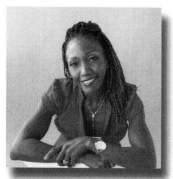

Kim Farmer is the CEO of Mile High Fitness & Wellness, a corporate wellness organization serving companies of all sizes.

She has successfully helped companies integrate holistic wellness programming into the workplace by helping them reduce stress levels, improve performance, and productivity.

Her presentations inspire motivation and creativity, helping individuals make lasting, intrinsic behavior change using preventive wellness efforts.

Her energy unites teams and leaders, encouraging culture change using creative wellness programming.

She is a regular contributor to several media outlets, including print and radio, and has published books, articles, and DVDs.

"The human body is the best picture of the human soul."
~ Tony Robbins ~

Tampa, Florida, USA

Website: www.milehighfitness.com

Social Media:
- www.facebook.com/milehighfitness
- ww.linkedin.com/in/milehighfitness
- www.twitter.com/milehighfitness

Visit website for free consultation www.milehighfitness.com/getfit

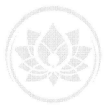

Wellness at Work:
Don't Just Sit There!

An Arabian proverb says, "He who has health has hope and he who has hope has everything." Nothing about having money, or cars, or even chocolate (my personal everything). Nope! Just your health.

Most of us work in an environment where social norms have led to us sitting all day. This has been one thing that has led to more of us being overweight, which then leads to other problems.

After working for corporate America for far too long, I realized I couldn't stand one more dull, meaningless, monotonous meeting and decided to take back my life! Well … I got laid off, but I still took my life back! It was probably the best decision I could have made. I mean, really, how many meetings does it take to make a decision?

Not to mention the following things were happening:

- I found myself 'sneaking' away from my desk to take walks during the day
- I would want to exercise at my desk but felt weird about doing it
- I would try to leave a early to catch the sunlight to play tennis after work
- My butt was getting wider. And wider. And wider

This was obviously a runaway train to me getting fat, sick, and even more unhappy. I was always thinking about things that I could do to get more movement during the work day since it was composed primarily of sitting at a desk. If any of this sounds familiar, keep reading.

I began to investigate what it would take to start teaching fitness classes. I imagined myself up there on stage, wearing my pink leotard and flipping my hair back in the wind while barking out orders. It became the most important thing to accomplish and I was determined that if I could just teach fitness classes (in my leotard), then my bucket list would be complete. So I studied, practiced, took the exam, and bam! Just like that I became a Jane Fonda wannabe. Ok a very dark skinned Jane, but I did it! I then went on to get certified as a personal trainer and a host of other things I won't bore you with.

It became quite obvious to me, and a lot of other people, the workplace was like a virtual host for weight gain, disease, and a general unhealthy culture. Luckily, I wasn't the only one who realized that since many of my first clients came from people who wanted fitness and nutrition classes at work. I wasn't sure exactly how the classes would be received by leadership teams in the workplace, but what did I have to lose?

It became my mission to help as many people as I could by bringing healthy programs to their location. At the time, this idea wasn't brand new, but certainly not as common as it is today. Back then, most companies felt like they had a wellness program if they had a newsletter and an apple on the front desk. Back then, entire comprehensive programs were only afforded to large corporations while small companies were generally unable to afford effective programs.

According to the Centers for Disease Control, workplace health programs are defined as: 'a coordinated and comprehensive set of health promotion and protection strategies implemented at the worksite that includes programs, policies, benefits, environmental supports, and links to the surrounding community designed to encourage the health and safety of all employees.'

At that time I didn't really know this but I knew I couldn't allow things to continue the way they were with insurance costs increasing 55% since 2008 and 20% since 2013. Unreal right? This is in some ways due to chronic illnesses and the medication required to treat them, but I also think its just plain business.

I knew prevention was the answer and prescription medication was not. I knew I wouldn't be able to 'cure' everyone, but maybe I could help one person and that one person mattered. I put on my pink cape (that matched my leotard) and set out on a quest to save the world!

As I started to get more knowledgeable on the topic of wellness at work, I realized the industry had been through quite a few changes over the years. Technically, wellness at work programs started in the early to mid-90s with c-level executives receiving access to personal trainers right in their office. Yep, the rest of us were left to our own devices and donuts while those that were well paid received the concierge level treatment.

Employee Assistance Programs (EAP) came on the scene in order to help with alcohol and drug dependencies. This was great at the time, but unfortunately it created a stigma that if you used the EAP services, you were a crackhead.

EAPs have evolved greatly over the years to include many services, including; fitness and nutrition coaching for some, but the utilization is very low, only around 5%. This is very unfortunate since according to NAMI [1], 2.4 million adults have schizophrenia, 6.1 million adults have bipolar disorder, and 6.9 million adults have major depression. These numbers aren't including teens or children. Many wellness programs are beginning to include more options for employees wanting to improve their state of mental health, however, I believe it may take some work to increase the utilization of these and EAP programs to show a positive impact on company culture.

Regardless of the program offered at work, the responsibility of your level of health starts with you. Unless you are someone who always does what is recommended by your employer, then you may choose not to participate in your companies' wellness program (if there is one), get your annual physical, eat nutritious foods everyday, etc. So while your employer may do its very best to provide you all the resources you could ever need to obtain higher levels of health, consider that a bonus (if it is offered) and make it a priority to improve your habits as soon as possible.

Moving at Work

For some people, even the thought of exercising causes anxiety. Perhaps you don't fall into this extreme category but for some, they have started and stopped a routine so many times they lost count. Trying something over and over again with little to no results can cause anyone to have a low level of confidence when it comes to trying it one more time.

However, I have good news! You don't have to exercise, you only have to move. That's all. Just move. Easy right?

One of the worst things you can do is to sit at your desk all day at work and not move. Your metabolism slows down after so much sitting which means you are burning less calories throughout the day making it harder to maintain a healthy weight. You burn about 50 calories more per hour simply by standing which can add up! So if you can, get up from your desk every so often (preferably once an hour) and just do something for about 10 minutes. This could be taking a walk around the office, marching in place, dancing at your desk (not on it or you might catch a few dollar bills), or doing a few sit/stands in your chair. Whatever you can do with the space you have is fine. Just don't sit there for an hour straight.

Force yourself to move for at least 10 minutes. If you are lucky and have a gym at work, consider yourself very lucky. If your company allows you an hour for lunch, that's a perfect time to move for 30 minutes. Don't be like me and watch your butt get wider.

Eating at Work

This could be a chapter in itself! I'll do my best to highlight some practical things that could help you make a plan to choose wisely when you are at work.

If you have a desk job, proper nutrition is imperative for you in order to maintain your weight and overall health status. Your metabolism is highly dependent on your activity level and it tends to slow down more when you aren't doing anything to help it run throughout the day. If you don't have much movement throughout the day, then you need to take control of your nutrition.

This doesn't have to be anything complicated, and most importantly, it must not be a complete overhaul from your current eating plan. Whether or not you think you have a plan, you do. The lack of a plan is the presence of a plan by default. The plan is to not to have one. So it's time to make one on purpose.

Start by making enough of the things you like to eat in advance, enough to bring to work for a few days during the week. Whatever you make at home is more than likely going to be somewhat more nutritious than going out for a quick run at lunch. Start modifying the things you like slightly by adding more fruit or veggies, lean protein, and complex carbs. Eventually you will naturally crave foods with more nutrition which is (in my opinion) the way it should be.

Our bodies were created to thrive off of plant food, and if you give it a chance, you will crave it more than other foods.

There is no magic answer- everyone has a different lifestyle, preferences, schedule, etc., so your plan will likely be different than everyone else. The key is to figure out what works best for you, and then do that.

I hope this information has been helpful. My organization has created a way to bring activities to the workplace to help make it a little easier. Please stay connected with me; I can't wait to hear your comments and feedback!

"All the money in the world can't buy you back good health."
~ Reba McEntire ~

Dr. Karen Valentin

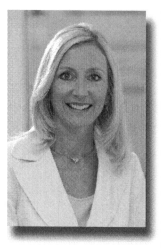

Dr. Karen Valentin specialized in Physics and Atmospheric Sciences at Drexel U. in Philadelphia and completed her dissertation in Natural Sciences in Mainz, Germany.

She worked as an environmental consultant before resigning after her second of four children was born.

Top priority for over a decade was child-rearing, especially since one of her children has mental disabilities.

Initially working from home, she developed an expertise in nutrition, health, and fitness areas.

In 2012 she opened her own consulting practice med. BodyForming in Mannheim.

Through *Unicity*, she has expanded her business with independent partners in over 6 countries and aims to "Make Life Better".

"It doesn't matter what happens to us in life.
It is how we deal with what happens to us in life
that determines where we're going to go."
~ Bob Proctor ~

Mannheim, Baden-Wurttemberg, Germany

Website: www.med-body-forming.de

Social Media:
- www.facebook.com/MedBodyForming/
- www.linkedin.com/in/dr-karen-valentin-health-coach/
- www.xing.com/profile/Karen_Valentin

Contact Karen with your comments and questions in English or German. info@med-body-forming.de

Do's and Don'ts for Caregivers of Mentally Disabled People

For anybody with a close family member with mental disabilities, family life can be an enormous challenge. 'Life isn't fair' is a good fact to keep in mind when confronted with a family member developing, or born with, mental disabilities.

How can you cope? Who can be of outside help? What future lies ahead for the person with mental disabilities? What measures should be taken to give them the best chances of a fulfilled and happy life? How can you successfully meet the best interests of each family member to have a pleasant family life together?

My personal experience as mother of a child with special needs extends over 23 years and certainly caught me by surprise; I was unprepared. My second of four children was born in 1996 with fine scores and no apparent disabilities. Her initial development was not obviously delayed, and her difficult behavior as a two-year-old I put to the "terrible twos" all parents know about.

At the age of three, she had her first obvious partial-complex epilepsy attack and I was suddenly catapulted into the world of severe neurological diseases and developmental problems. Coming from a family of academics and married to an oral surgeon, I had never envisioned one of my children not finishing college, let alone not managing the regular kindergarten, and grade school programs. Determining which medication and which therapeutic training would best help my daughter reach optimal health became my top priorities. There were many clinics to choose from, and fortunately, one nearby therapeutic center for young children like my daughter.

Making the right selections, listening to the right advice, and maintaining hope and a pleasant family life as much as possible were all imperative to the welfare of the whole family.

My sources of strength and moral support during the toughest years (1999-2005) were our extended family, my circle of friends, our babysitters, and my husband who backed me up and provided the financial support for our family.

Neurologists and pediatricians provided the main expertise regarding selection of my daughter's medication and treatments. I had my daughter checked by specialists at one neuropediatric center in the U.S. and at five centers in Germany where we live. My daughter's developmental progress in many areas can be accredited to excellent special education teachers and specialists in behavior and cognitive therapy, physical therapy, neurofeedback, speech therapy, and equine therapy. Her exceptionally patient special education teachers over 13 years of schooling enabled my daughter to reach much higher reading and writing skills than experts predicted.

Based on my experiences, I am sharing the following guidelines for other caregivers. Some apply most to the acute phase, when the mental disability either suddenly manifests itself or becomes significantly worse, while others are relevant for the long-term caregiving phases:

Top priority is the accurate diagnosis and medical therapy for the affected person.

This can be a long process, however, other important parts of family life cannot be ignored for extended periods. With many mental disabilities, there is no absolute cure. So the best options of treatment with minimal side effects need to be considered. Often the cause of the neurological problem is unknown. In such cases, new genetic analyses could perhaps provide valuable information.

Don't try to do the professional therapy or special education yourself.

At some point during the first critical years with my daughter, I found the sound advice not to be both "Mother" and "Teacher" or "Therapist". The experts have been specially trained and are paid to do the grinding work needed to help people with mental disabilities gain or regain more capabilities, or better behavior. It is enough to be Mother or Father. Providing the best home with a loving atmosphere for the whole family is what we need to do primarily.

Don't resign to bad predictions of therapists or doctors.

Professional evaluations of the present state are important, but predictions can prove wrong. In the case of my daughter, at the age of six, she took a series of neurological and developmental tests at a renowned clinic with an experienced neuropsychologist. I was told she was so impaired she would not likely ever be able to read much more than a stop sign.

At that moment I was crushed, yet unwilling to accept that dismal future for my daughter. Had I resigned to that evaluation, I wouldn't have done everything in my power to give her the most therapy possible and ensure her acceptance into an inclusive school with special education teachers working alongside regular teachers.

Much to the surprise of the neuropsychologist, my daughter's reading skills skyrocketed by the age of 13.

Today at the age of 23, she regularly reads the news in two languages on her notebook or cell phone. She has perfect intonation in English and German, and is highly entertaining to her listeners. This competency allows her to follow her favorite sports teams, music groups, and celebrities; which she thoroughly enjoys. Have I made my point?

Have courage to accept the challenge of caregiving.

My husband and I opted to have our daughter attend a day-school program and never sent her away for overnight schooling or treatments. Our daughter's thorough integration in our family has proven beneficial to each of us.

Do not neglect your own health, nutrition and general welfare.

It is important to maintain a healthy diet, get regular exercise, and get seven or more hours of sleep each night. The recently discovered strong relationship between the gut, the brain, and our emotions demonstrates the need to maintain a healthy gut with a fiber-rich diet containing lots of phytonutrients, low on sugar, high on protein, and healthy fats. While occasional party or "comfort" food and beverages are acceptable, long-term eating and drinking habits need to be responsible. The caregiver needs to stay fit to be of service, and it is vital to prevent the onset of other health disorders, like type 2 diabetes. Sport options for people with special needs may be limited, but home DVDs with aerobics and dance exercises were my daughter's top choices for years.

Practice of meditation or mindfulness is recommended.

I had my regular prayers and time of relaxation in the garden or elsewhere to help me relax and regain my peace of mind. My daughter enjoys our daily prayers and "chills" listening to music.

Neglecting the other family members is not an option.

My oldest son was two years old when his sister came along and had little patience for her and her misbehavior for many years. While he demanded and deserved to have equal attention, as did his other siblings born later, common playtime and family activities improved social skills of everybody in the family.

Keep a good sense of humor.

People with mental disabilities should never be laughed at, but laughing with them about something humorous is good fun. My daughter sometimes says the funniest things and is intentionally witty. It is a pleasure having her around.

In conclusion, I hope you gained insight on how to master the challenges of caregiving for people with mental disabilities. Life isn't fair, but each life bears more riches than we can imagine.

*"Never believe that a few caring people can't change the world.
For, indeed, that's all who ever have."*
~ Margaret Mead ~

Marquita h Catallo-Madruga

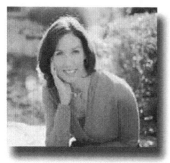

Dr. Marci graduated from Regis University with a Doctorate in Physical Therapy in May of 2005.

She has served populations from low income to professional athletes and everything in-between.

She truly enjoys spending time with her clients and getting to know them.

Marci believes that the whole person is part of the injury picture, not just the current complaint they may have.

She wanted to make sure she was getting to each patient in a one-to-one relationship and help them "get right" so they could go back to whatever activity they were previously doing.

Marci and her husband, Daniel, are originally from California. Marci and her Husband were blessed with twin boys in late Summer 2010. Alex and Austin are a huge joy and a huge handful.

"Disease mongering has lead to poorer health in the country"
~ R. Moynhin ~

Centennial, Colorado, USA

Website: www.5280restorativemed.com

Social Media:
- www.facebook.com/agilityphysio
- www.instagram.com/agilityphysicaltherapy
- www.youtube.com/channel/UCL-j3h9jL8jeXNxQJJbmzvw

Please contact us for more information drmarci@agilityphysio.com

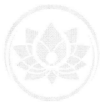

Restorative Health:
Be Connected To Our Body and Mind

"While there is evidence to support that the natural environment leads to improvements in health markers, more evidence is needed to show what disease may benefit and why."[1]

As a person living in the 21st century, I am often confounded by the significant lack of health I am surrounded by. It seems people are less connected to the environment and to the people around them than they are to their devices. We have stopped relying on our true person-to-person connections and moved to a world where we could go a full day without uttering a word to another human.

If you type in a search for the effects of electronic devices on health, the results are kind of scary. This chapter will focus on restorative health and how we can get back to the last time our body agreed it could do what we asked of it. Restorative health is very individualized and takes a commitment from the person and the provider. It makes sure both parties are invested to obtain the best outcomes for all involved.

For the last decade, I have been looking for ways to restore my health back to the way it was pre-kids. The things I am looking for are: sleep, workout recovery, feeling comfortable in my body, less seasonal allergies, and less pain. I sought out the help of a physician in 2012 and was directed through a medical model that wanted to drug away my symptoms and maybe (definitely) cause some other symptoms. It was not the root cause of what was happening, it was a band aid approach. Cover-ups don't work. They simply push the problem to a higher level while partially masking it. What I discovered was that I had a bunch of food allergies that came back full force while pregnant and were wreaking havoc on my body. You see, true health starts from within, and from the environment around you.

Inflammation occurs when you take in foods you have sensitivities and allergies too. Inflammation starts in the mouth, continues to the esophagus, leads to the stomach, and ends in the gut through to the colon.

The digestive tract is of utmost importance in our health because it is where 90% of the nutrients we take in each day are absorbed. Think of this area of your body similar to the skin, with a severe bug bite. That bug bite becomes inflamed, itchy, swells more, you usually agitate it further, and it perpetuates the problem. The same is true of the digestive system. If you have a sunburn, how healthy is your skin at the time when it is tight, dry, and peeling? Does it absorb lotion well or just appear dry and irritated a few hours later?

If you are causing inflammation due to food sensitivities and allergies, what does the digestive tract look like and how does it feel? One of the problems we have as a society is if I can't see it, it must not be real. I can ignore it and it will go away, or I can take something for it. This "disease mongering" is part of the pharmaceutical industry push to sell drugs that should likely not be on the market, but also add to the symptoms you experience because they cover a health issue with a "band-aid."

The discipline to restore your health has to come from with-in, but I believe one must also have support. That support can be a health coach, physician, family member, or trusted friends. The non-coach or physician should be someone willing to truly push you and not damage the relationship. The accountability from them must be true to your desire for health. It works best if they are trying to get back some measure of health as well.

The typical start of restoring health happens through doing a series of blood work and allergy testing. The best thing about this is that a lot of allergies now can be tested via hair sample, blood work, mouth scraping, and/or spit collection. The patch testing is still an option, but you can find cheaper, less invasive means through online labs.

Once you find the things that are causing you inflammation on a daily basis, we tailor an elimination diet to those sensitivities. The elimination diet process is no less than 90 days. If you feel you have extreme or severe food allergies and sensitivities, it may be recommended for six months. This is so the digestive tract has a chance to heal. If it is still "sunburned" it can not absorb nutrients.

The next step is to look at stool samples and find weaknesses in the microbiome and support them. Hormone testing may also be done to look at imbalances and supplements recommended for support.

With the elimination diet, we focus a lot on the patterns of sleep. Sleep has been discussed a lot over the last decade as a major player in health. There is research to support the fact that lack of sleep causes your body to become insulin resistant, increasing your chances of diabetes. It can lead to stroke due to increased blood pressure, adrenal fatigue, thyroid dysfunction, and weight gain.

Sleep is when your body truly restores itself. Most of the repair work done is during the time when you are sleeping. Your body goes through a significant amount of detoxification while sleeping. If you look through the *Chinese Medicine Body Clock* for organ detoxification, you can see the detoxification of the liver and the gallbladder occur between 11:00 PM and 1:00 AM.

Going to bed and sleep at a regular time also decreases the likelihood of insomnia and sleep disorders. There has been evidence to show that stopping technology device use; like television and dimming lights in the areas of the house you will be in 30 minutes prior to bedtime will improve your ability to fall asleep quickly.

We typically recommend both food and sleep journal. These journals should include what you ate, whether it was protein, carbohydrate, or fruit and veggies; the time that you ate, and how much water you drink. It should also include any activity done in the day and your general feeling at the beginning and ending of each day based on mood and stress level. The sleep journal should include what time you went to bed, if you fell asleep easily; if you woke up what time was it; how you felt in the morning when waking up.

Restoring your health also includes periods of time outside, unconnected from the digital world. A four year longitudinal study in the UK showed that people who had access to green space had lower incidence of disease, particularly cardiovascular and psychological.

We encourage mindfulness during this time in the outside world. We ask for people to focus on how they currently feel, then change to how they want to feel that day or moment. We then ask them to say four positive affirmations on the type of feeling they want to have that day in relationship to work, home, body image, and health overall. For instance: "I enjoy working with each one of my clients. At home I am working well to encourage positive homework behaviors in my children. I am my perfect self every day and I am gaining control over my back pain each moment."

Restoring your health is a process that will likely take 18-months to three years, depending on the amount of damage that has occurred over time. We hope that your journey is fulfilling and guides you to a better place in your life.

Luanne Nelson

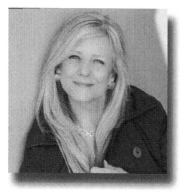

Luanne Nelson is a #1 Bestselling Author, motivational speaker, and certified health coach through the MacDonald Center for Obesity Prevention and Education (COPE) & M. Louise Fitzpatrick College of Nursing at Villanova University.

She encourages men and women to learn new skills to attain healthier lifestyles.

Luanne understands the importance of nurturing the body, soul, and spirit to achieve optimal fitness and has had the privilege of coaching men and women all over the USA.

She studied English Literature at Westminster College in PA and Journalism at Marquette University in WI.

Luanne offers a practical health program and loves to help her clients attain their personally tailored health goals.

"Nature gives you the face you have at twenty;
it's up to you to merit the face you have at fifty."
~ Coco Chanel ~

Milwaukee, Wisconsin, USA

Website: www.LuanneNelson.com

Social Media:
- www.facebook.com/luanne.nelson.healthcoach
- www.linkedin.com/in/luanne-nelson-b8599047

If you would like a program that is simple, sustainable, and affordable, please contact me! InfoAllAboutYou@gmail.com

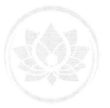

Aging Gracefully

Time flies! Navigating through the sixth decade of life, I've had plenty of time to learn from my mistakes, I've also had enough time to get a few things right. I hope you'll find a few of the highlights I've included here to be worth implementing into your own life.

If you're younger and reading this, maybe you'll gather some useful info on how not to look like a train wreck by the time you turn 60. If you are in your 60s (like I am), I hope you'll be able to relate to some of the tips, maybe finding a few useful new tips. Age allows for wisdom; experience is a great teacher.

> *"We all sorely complain of the shortness of time,*
> *and yet have much more than we know what to do with.*
> *Our lives are either spent in doing nothing at all,*
> *or in doing nothing to the purpose, or in doing nothing that we ought to do.*
> *We are always complaining that our days are few,*
> *and acting as though there would be no end of them."*
> *~ Lucius Annaeus Seneca ~*

Every day counts. As a certified health coach, I love working together with men and women to achieve health goals. Truth is, I've always been a "health nut." More than thirty years ago, I was one of "those" moms who made my children's baby food from scratch. I steamed, mashed, and baked whole foods several times a day for years. Throughout my life, a passion for fitness and healthy living has been a constant.

Aging is a fact of life, looking like an ancient mess is optional

Seventy-eight years is the average lifespan in this country according to the Center for Disease Control and Prevention. I think it's safe to say that we all wonder from time to time: What can I do to live longer, feel good, and look better while I progress through life into a ripe old age?

Scientists have found that long-lived individuals have little in common with one another in education, income, or profession. The similarities they do share, however, reflect their lifestyles—many are nonsmokers, are not obese, and cope well with stress[1]. Point being, good health is not a new exercise routine, a diet, or any other one thing, it's a lifestyle.

Healthful Habits Reap Rewards

Over the years, I've randomly asked dozens of healthy, attractive older people their secret for aging gracefully. Almost everyone shared the same answers.

> "Pay attention to what you're doing!"
> "Life is precious and it goes by fast."
> "Time stops for no one."
> "Don't get upset over the small stuff."
> "Choose your battles wisely!"

All good advice. I am going to add this: "Brush your teeth and floss regularly." I'm married to a dentist who has drilled into my psyche the dangerous link between challenged teeth and heart disease.

Have you noticed most people usually don't pay attention to their well-being until well into adulthood? A few extra pounds might trigger a diet, maybe even a temporary exercise program; perhaps a different day will call for stretching and jogging a few laps around the block.

Half-measures availed us nothing. I've learned developing good habits requires constancy, paying attention and doing things on purpose, even when we don't feel like it. Dare I say, good habits require discipline.

We all know the importance of getting enough sleep, washing our hands before eating, doing unto others as you would have done unto you. We all learn how to share from our hearts, how to make new friends, how to nurture relationships. We learn how to celebrate life, how to forgive ourselves, how to truly love. We also all know eating broccoli once a year is not going to change a thing.

So, let's explore a few other things I've learned we should be doing on purpose.

Preserve Your Body

Our bodies are what we are given to wear in this lifetime. To take care of your skin, start with staying well-hydrated. No, a cup of coffee does not count as a cup of water. Remember to moisturize your skin, too. My grandmother shared this tidbit with me when I was a little girl: "Always keep your face clean, occasionally using witch hazel on a cotton ball to get rid of any excess dirt." She told me to skip foundation, advising, "Let your face breathe." She shared her thoughts with me that American women wear too much makeup and do not take care of their skin. Since she had beautiful skin, I listened to her. To this day, I mix a little witch hazel with some vitamin E oil to use as an anti-aging serum in my beauty routine.

Enjoy several smaller meals a day instead of three large ones. Our bodies respond well when we "graze," providing fuel periodically throughout the day. I've been known to bake a small potato, bag it and put it in my purse for a mid-afternoon snack. A handful of pistachios is heaven for your heart. They're little roto-rooters for your arteries.

It's important to feed your brain, too. Every day, learn something new. Years ago, my children brought something new they learned that day to the dinner table. Learn, on purpose, they learned how to adjust attitudes, set boundaries, set goals, and how to make lists to achieve goals. Go out and buy yourself a paper calendar and a notebook. It's old school, I know, but there is something rewarding about crossing things off of a list.

A Sense of Humor is Important

Plan ahead. When I was in my twenties, old age and dying really did not cross my mind; I think at that age we believe our skin will stay taut and glow forever. Wrong. That cute little boobie tat of a butterfly you are thinking of getting? Think again. It's going to look like a deranged, rabid bat in a few decades. Just don't do it. Also, remember that paper calendar and notebook I just suggested you buy? I am still not convinced my computer is dependable enough to keep track of my life. There is something disconcerting about having my life saved on a cloud somewhere. Learn to laugh at yourself.

Nourish Your Spirit

Celebrate your emotions. It's alright to be angry, sad, jealous, scared, bored, anxious; it's what we do with our feelings that's important. Create beautiful places to relax. Learn how to be dignified in failure. Read the Ten Commandments and follow them the best you can every day.

Remember, what comes out of your mouth is as important as what goes in it. The tongue can be used as a deadly sword. Be careful with it. There is joy and there is crashing disappointment.

Call your Mom and your Dad. You don't have to love them. You don't even have to like them. They did, however, bring your lovely life into this universe. So, say hello to them once in a while. Be nice. Believe in Miracles.

A few final gems...

Develop an attitude of gratitude. Make a list of things you're grateful for and carry it around in your back pocket. Go talk to someone who has been around for several decades – there's a lot to be said for wisdom gained from experience. Remember, there are support groups for everything from overeating to learning how to work through the loss of a living adult child.

Say one nice thing to a total stranger every day. Stretch. Bend. Be a person of substance, strength, and conviction with an open mind ready to change if new evidence is compelling enough. Walk. A short, daily walk clears your mind and improves your mood. Apologize right away when wrong; even if the apology is not accepted. Keep your side of the street clean. What others think of you is none of your business. Breathe. Adopt a cause. Stand up straight. Seek the Truth. Always, seek the Truth.

Remember, good health is a lifestyle. Nurture your mind, your body and your spirit. Go forth and age gracefully!

"We don't stop playing because we grow old;
we grow old because we stop playing."
~ George Bernard Shaw ~

Alexis Dowd

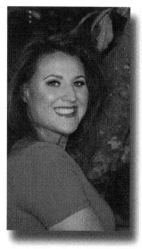

Alexis Dowd is a qualified EFT practitioner, Matrix Re-imprinting practitioner and Angelic Usui Reiki Master who specialises in emotional and mental healing.

She's also a wellbeing devotee who believes in freedom of choice and that health and wellbeing is unique to everyone.

She is the co-founder of *Wellbeing Umbrella* where we connect wellness seekers to a world full of options to enhance individual, and workplace wellness, while providing support to those practitioners and professionals who want to make a difference too.

"You must be the change that you wish to see in the world."
~ Mahatma Gandhi ~

Wigan, Greater Manchester, United Kingdom

Website: www.wellbeingumbrella.com

Social Media:
- www.facebook.com/wellbeingumbrella
- www.instagram.com/wellbeingumbrella
- www.facebook.com/wellbeingumbrellabusiness

Access my FREE eBook tapping script for anger; includes tapping points and process, and monthly wisdom. http://bit.ly/WellbeingUmbrellaEFTresource

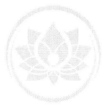

EFT – What Is It & How Does It Work?

How I came to be a qualified EFT (emotional freedom techniques) practitioner was somewhat a means to an end; in order for me to gain a qualification in another therapy it was a requirement to pass my certification in EFT first.

I'd previously done lots of inner work using the law of attraction, gratitude journaling. and positive affirmations. So when I was presented with tapping techniques that, in the first round or two, touched on negative statements, I felt uncomfortable tapping. However, several months after my training I met fellow EFT practitioner, Veronica, who completely changed how I felt about EFT and showed me just how powerful this technique is.

Veronica conducted a private one-to-one EFT session to alleviate my fear of public speaking. I'd been asked numerous times to do presentations and talks but I was crippled by fear. This was due to experiences I had suffered during primary and secondary school, which had always remained with me.

Whilst working on my fear of public speaking, traumas resurfaced that had occurred in my younger years which I had never spoken about to anyone, nor dealt with.

The powerful thing about EFT is even though you may not be working on an issue directly, it can bring up what needs to be worked on, what needs to be released and healed to allow you to move forward. After seeing the huge change in my life, my passion to share these techniques with others was immense. I learned the only way to heal the dark pains of the past is to shine a light on them so that they can dissolve.

EFT is often referred to as "psychological acupressure". It works by releasing blockages within the energy system that are the source of emotional intensity and distress. Having these blockages in our energy system, in addition to challenging us emotionally, can lead to limiting beliefs, behaviours, and an inability to feel fulfilled.

Acupressure, acupuncture, and reflexology all work in the same way: pressure is applied to specific points on the meridians (or ends of meridians) to clear blockages in the body's energy channels, allowing the energy to flow freely.

EFT is a healing process that can provide remarkable results for emotional, performance, and physical issues (including chronic pain) in just one session. Through tapping, you can experience some profound changes in both your emotional and physical wellbeing. It's a valuable tool which can be used in everyday life, especially when dealing with emotions such as anger, frustration, distress, or worry.

Within 5-10 minutes of tapping you can feel totally different about the situation and can proceed with clarity. How many times have you reacted in the heat of the moment? And later come to regret it? EFT gives you the opportunity to release the intense emotion and respond accordingly from a clear space.

Tapping teddy bears are wonderful when working with children or teenagers, especially if they are prone to outbursts of anger, suffer from anxiety, have trouble communicating, and/or find it difficult to express themselves.

When I'm delivering presentations on EFT to a large group, to allow them to experience just how quickly and how amazing EFT is, I usually pick the subject of anger, because it's an emotion that when speaking to large groups, 99% of the audience will have experienced; for example, a situation that has made them angry in the past. Whereas if I chose to speak about anxiety maybe only 50% of the audience will be able to participate and feel the shift.

Here's how it works.

There are 4 steps to the Tapping process:

Step 1 – Using an Intensity Scale of 1-10

Choose a topic or issue and, if you can, name the emotion attached to the topic.
- Example – I'm so annoyed with my partner.
- What's the emotion behind it? Anger, embarrassment, fear, overwhelm, etc.?
- Rate the intensity of your feelings about the topic/issue on a scale of 1-10.
- 1 is feeling fine and 10 is extremely intense.

Step 2 – Set-up Statement: This Step Is Very Important

- It's made up of 2 parts
  (first part is the issue, which is usually negative; ... second part is something positive to 'lift' and balance the phrase).
- 1st part: You always start with 'Even though ....'
- EXAMPLE – Even though I am annoyed with my partner...
- 2nd part: I deeply and completely accept myself.
- Why it's significant. This is to align the conscious with the subconscious.

Step 3 – The Sequence of Tapping Points

- We start off tapping and talking about the issue (which is negative).
- We then tap and talk about wanting to look at the issue in a different way.
- We want to let it go, we want to find another way of looking at it.
- Moving through to tap and talk in a positive and uplifting way.

Step 4 – Repeat Step 1

- Check in with yourself, where are you now on the intensity scale?
- Have you remained the same or have you gone down?

Now, Let's Tap!

Use your fingertips on specific acupressure points. It doesn't matter if you wish to use two fingers, three, or four. You can swap hands during the tapping rounds should your arm become tired. You may see many different ways to tap on the internet, none work better than any other, they're all fabulous.

Think of an issue that has made you angry, this could be a situation that happened three years ago or just this morning. Close your eyes and go with the first subject that comes to mind. You want to pick an issue that has an intensity rating of 5 or above, anything below is not really an issue.

- It could be you had a heated argument with a family member that's caused a family rift and you no longer communicate.
- Someone cut in front of you whilst driving this morning.
- You're being blamed for something you didn't do.
- You're feeling justice wasn't carried out.

It could be absolutely anything!

Start with the set-up statement whilst tapping on the side of your hand (karate chop point): 'Even though I have 'this issue' I deeply and completely accept myself'. Repeat this statement three times whilst tapping continuously on the karate chop point.

Then continue by tapping on each point, e.g. eyebrow point, 5 -7 times.

Tapping Script for Anger

Round One:

Eyebrow Point (EB): All this anger.
Side of the Eye (SE): I have so much anger.
Under the Eye (UE): I'm so full of anger right now.
Under the Nose (UN): It's in every part of me.
Under the Mouth (UM): I'm so full of anger.
Collarbone (CB): I can feel it in every cell of my body.
Under the Arm (UA): I feel it in my bones and in my gut.
Top of the Head (TH): I can even feel it in my heart.

> EB: I am so furious right now.
> SE: I am absolutely fuming.
> UE: I have every right to be angry about this.
> UN: This person/situation has me so angry right now.
> UM: This feeling is so strong.
> CB: I want to release it, but I don't really want to release it.
> UA: I am justified in my anger.
> TH: I have every right to be angry!!

> EB: It's okay to feel angry.
> SE: I give myself permission to feel this anger.
> UE: I'm moving through it now.
> UN: This situation is not okay with me.
> UM: But I choose to feel calmer about it.
> CB: I'm willing to start letting go of this anger.
> UA: Maybe not all of it.
> TH: But at least a little bit of it.

EB: I'm willing to feel calmer now.
SE: I'm willing to release this tension in my body.
UE: I'm willing to breathe easier now.
UN: I'm willing to start feeling peaceful again.
UM: I'm willing to calm down and relax my body.
CB: I'm willing to feel okay again.
UA: I'm willing to dissolve this remaining anger.
TH: I'm willing to take control of my thoughts and feelings.

EB: I am a strong, intelligent and capable person.
SE: I choose to control my feelings.
UE: I choose to let go of this anger.
UN: Knowing it'll benefit me.
UM: I choose to feel peace and calm.
CB: I choose to breathe easy and let go this tension in body.
UA: I choose to feel better.
TH: I am feeling better now.

Now just take a nice deep breath and relax.

How do you feel? Check in with yourself, where are you now on the intensity scale? Has the number come down?

In rare cases the number can increase before it comes down, this is typically because you may feel you're only at a number 5 or 6 but when you start tapping you realise that the situation is more intense than you first thought. Keep tapping until you bring the number to at least a 1 or 2, this can usually be achieved within 10 minutes.

Please do not use EFT to tap through any serious traumas on your own, this can become overwhelming and intense and should be conducted by a qualified EFT practitioner only.

Reina Rose

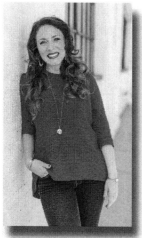

Wellness and abundance expert, Reina Rose, has dedicated her life to uncovering insights into true mind, body, and soul wellness and abundance.

Since first launching her business in 2003, she has progressed from teaching wellness and abundance workshops, to leading immersive life transformative retreats that help high performance individuals temporarily pause so they may realign with their true values and reengage more peacefully and effectively.

Bringing greater peace and prosperity to the world one influencer at a time is Reina's life mission.

Reina also helps cultivate spiritual, emotional, and financial abundance for communities throughout the globe with her writing, teaching, and service in churches and orphanages.

"Come to Me, all you who are weary and burdened, and I will give you rest."
~ Jesus in Matthew 11:28 ~

Flagstaff, Arizona, USA

Website: www.reina-rose.com

Social Media:
- www.linkedin.com/in/reina-rose-b95488183/
- www.instagram.com/reina_rose_wellness/
- www.facebook.com/Reina-Rose-Wellness-387797905412590/

Join Reina's life transforming retreats. Rest and break down barriers to abundance in your life! www.reina-rose.com

Rest and Restore to Have More: Eight Steps to Avoid Burnout

Burnout is a word on everyone's lips these days. With the increasing demands of corporate environments, heavy workloads, and the lack of work-life balance, it is no wonder that people reporting symptoms of burnout is on the rise. The even more staggering concern may be those completely unconscious or unable to admit to burnout all together.

In the *Wall Street Journal* article "When Stress At Work Causes Drama At Home," it is reported that work is seeping into weekends and this spillover effect can jeopardize relationships [1]. The article explains that when a person comes home stressed from work, they are far more likely to express angry outbursts towards their loved ones, further perpetuating a downward spiral of stress both at work and at home. How do we put an end to this work-life stress cycle? I believe it is by creating space for restorative downtime.

We become our habits, so if we have habits of rushing out the door with a breakfast bar in hand, drinking loads of coffee to get through overbooked, overstressed days, only to take sleeping pills or consume alcohol to stop the day from spinning around in our minds at night, our mental, physical, and spiritual health will reflect those habits. However, if we choose to wake up with time to ease into the morning, carve out time for a mental pause throughout our day, and actually take advantage of the vacation time that has been piling up from years of working nonstop, our health will reflect a much nicer picture.

Oprah Winfrey speaks about one of her favorite golden retrievers, Gracie, who was always on the go. Never slowing down for anything. The most energetic of the three she had at the time, Gracie died from choking on a ball while playing fetch. Oprah described that instant she saw Gracie laying on the ground dead, she realized that if she didn't slow down, she would share the same fate. The good news is, we don't need to wait for a wakeup call to change our habits.

It is no secret that today's society is overworked, overstressed, malnourished, and unrested. We are constantly on the go, striving to do more, be more, and accomplish more. Which means, it is more imperative than ever to give the body, mind, and spirit the rest it needs. How does one do this and still get all the tasks completed on the ever increasing checklist of life? Luckily, studies show that taking restorative downtime actually increases our productivity.

An article on Forbes.com describes how something as simple as taking a dedicated lunch break instead of eating at your desk increases productivity, improves mental well-being, boosts creativity, and leads to more healthy habits [2].

Here are a few simple steps to destress and implement restorative downtime in your own life:

1. Re-Prioritize:

Ask yourself questions such as "If I could only work half the hours I work now, how could I get my work done?" "If I only had ten more years to live, how would I spend them?" or "What tasks can I delegate, automate, or eliminate altogether?" As you begin to eliminate tasks that do not require your expertise, you will begin to open up more mental space for your own creativity to flow. Do this both at work and at home for tasks that do not require your skills. For example, hiring a gardener or housekeeper may free up more time for you to spend with the kids, read a book, or take a yoga class.

2. Do One Thing At a Time:

There is so much research proving that multitasking is simply doing many things poorly. Focus on one task at a time, and give yourself some mental kudos for completing each task. Also, when it comes to meal times, put away electronic devices and allow yourself time to imagine possibilities, talk to a loved one, savor the food, and focus on digesting.

3. Take Breaks:

Not everyone has time for a week long retreat, but almost everyone has time to listen to a five minute guided meditation, step outside and put their feet on the earth for a few seconds, offer up a simple prayer, or even take a twenty minute power nap. When possible, it is so good for the soul to take longer pauses, whether it is for a weekend retreat or a two-week vacation to restore work-life balance.

4. Spend Time in Silence:

Time in silence and meditation has been shown to actually change the shape of our brains for the better. However, sitting in silence can be more challenging that it may seem. Beside being put on time-out as a child, many of us have gone our entire lives without practicing conscious silence. Try sitting in silence for ninety seconds. Begin by setting an intention in the form of a single word that speaks to you. For those who are religious, this could be the word "God," for others it could be something like "peace" or "calm." Once you are comfortable with ninety seconds, remain in silence for longer periods of time and see how your brain begins to change, making you more peaceful, calm, and patient even in your non-silent times.

5. Journal:

Writing has a very different effect on the brain than simply speaking something aloud. When we write down goals, statistics show an 80% increase in the likelihood of achieving them. Conversely, when we write our troubles down on paper, it is like dumping those problems into the pages and out of our brain for a while. A prayer journal is also a great tool for pouring out ones stresses to the Divine, however one may interpret that, and allowing the Divine mind to create peace and calm that leads to helpful solutions.

6. Sleep:

One of the symptoms of burnout is insomnia, however, it is so important for the average adult to get 7-9 hours of sleep. During sleep, blood flow increases to the brain and it is essentially cleansed in order to run smoothly for the following day. Another tip for making sleep most effective so the brain is properly cleansed, is to eat no less than four hours before bed. Eating within a few hours of going to sleep causes the blood to go to the stomach for digestion instead of the brain, taking precious blood flow away from restoring the brain at night.

7. Choose Different Thoughts:

Most people think the same thoughts, based on the past, and therefore experience the same reality. Instead of falling into the worst case scenario thinking, ask yourself questions such as "what would it take to have this circumstance turn out better than I could imagine?" And then allow the question to float around in your subconscious, allowing your intuition to discover answers over time. This practice of new thinking patterns will ultimately produce a new (and consciously chosen) reality. Making this a practice will heighten the serotonin and dopamine levels in your brain and alleviate stress.

8. Play Whenever Possible:

When we were kids we did not know the meaning of burnout. We knew what it meant to play and use our imagination. It was effortless. We weren't stressed. Find ways to incorporate play back into your life in whatever way that looks for you. Does that look like playing with your kids, your partner, joining the local kickball team or improv group? Doing something that allows you to feel carefree and playful will take that excess stress energy out of your body in a constructive way so that your family, friends, and co-workers do not receive the excess. It will also help maintain the mental, physical, and spiritual health balance.

However you choose to slow down and give yourself the restoration you require, it is imperative you choose these new habits intentionally. Prioritize time for yourself as a sacred practice or important appointment which you refuse to miss. Although it seems counter intuitive, taking time to slow down and nurture yourself is actually proven to make you much more effective, not to mention much more pleasant to spend time with!

How will you begin to create space for restorative downtime in your life? Write down some ideas, and begin implementing today!

"Contemplation is the highest form of activity."
~Aristotle ~

Jory Pradjinski

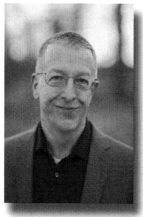

How we look at life matters. My choice was to either become bitter or become better.

"Why me" was changed to "why not me?"

I knew there were reasons for all I have been through. Some reasons came early, and some have not presented themselves yet.

For many years I felt a calling to help others. To reach out and give back from my journey.

In 2016 I founded the non-profit *Hope Instilled*. Our website, www.HopeInstilled.org, is a unique collection of information and resources.

Next, *Hope Against Pain* is the first action-based, peer-to-peer chronic pain support group.

In it I share the actual stages I went through to be alive today. We also offer actions each member can take in their own life. Bitter or better? The choice is yours.

"Healing doesn't mean the damage never existed.
It means the damage no longer controls our life."
~ Akshay Dubey ~

Milwaukee, Wisconsin, USA

Website: www.HopeInstilled.org

Social Media:
- www.facebook.com/HopeInstilled/
- www.linkedin.com/in/jorypradjinski
- www.twitter.com/hopeinstilled

Are you, or someone you know, living with chronic pain? We are an oasis from the darkness of pain. www.HopeInstilled.org

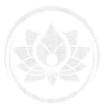

Facing the Monster While Being Completely Unaccepting

Pain is a monster which can devastate lives. It affects millions, yet no one wants to talk about it. Pain is an elephant in the room which society covers up with stigmas. Pain sits with another elephant covered up by society's stigmas, mental health. Alone they cause damage, together they devastate lives.

When the monster comes calling, your life will never be the same again. No one is safe from having pain come knocking on their door and moving in. Every person is an accident or an illness away from chronic pain. Everyone's chronic pain is a struggle, there is no competition for who has it worse.

For many years I was lost. Adrift in the darkness of chronic pain coming from many sources. Currently I have experienced over 30 traumas since injuring my back in 1987, when my life changed forever.

Life Changes Direction

I had been building my career in management within the automotive repair industry. At 26 years old, I was active and healthy. I never smoked and minimally drank alcohol. I was living my life. On August 27th, 1987 at 9:14am my world turned upside down. The day had begun like any other, a nice summer day at work. Or so I thought.

Two times per week we would receive a parts delivery which typically weighed between 200 - 300 pounds. We would manually remove the full crate from the delivery truck. That day was routine like any other. However, while moving the crate I felt a "pop" in my low back. It was one of those moments when you know something bad happened. Reluctantly, I began realizing this was a problem. In that split second from a work injury, my life began an unexpected journey. A doctor examination showed I had herniated my L5-S1 lumbar disc.

My pain journey included five back fusions in total due to three failed fusions. The surgery odyssey began in 1989. Each time I thought I could get on with my life, only to face yet another surgery. I didn't know if the repeated medical traumas would ever end. There were two follow-up procedures after finally achieving a solid fusion between my L5 vertebra and my sacrum (S1) in 1996.

In total, my lumbar back was cut open five times in the same scar tissue area. This resulted in nerve and muscle damage due to the repeated surgeries and the scar tissue build-up. The muscles on either side of the scar, about two inches wide in total, are non-responsive, essentially dead.

Life went on in ever worsening ways. Over time, the on-going, and increasing, chronic pain slowly ended relationships and my marriage. I felt more and more disconnected from life. The pain was an added challenge while raising two children. How much worse could life get for me? I would soon find out.

On a sunny afternoon in July of 2006, while at a stop light, I was rear-ended by an inattentive driver traveling approximately 50 mph, who never saw me. The injury results were cervical disc problems at C5-C6 and C6-C7; a severe concussion (the ninth in my life which I can remember) and I bruised the back of my skull from impacting the headrest during the thrashing my body endured. Just the week before I began wearing my seat belt all the time.

Just 5 years prior to this accident I had survived an 18-month period of suicidal ideation. Now I had even more challenges to my physical and mental health. How much becomes too much for one to take? My concentration began to fail me. The chronic pain continued to worsen from my back and now neck and head injuries. This has to be the worst it can get, I thought.

In January of 2013, I tripped on an electrical cord at home and fell face forward which dislodged my L4 vertebra. I thought my world had ended; this accident was too much to bear. I cannot take it anymore. I wanted off this horror ride. Yet, after a few months, the vertebra went back in place and I was referred to a chiropractor.

This horrific event started me on a miraculous journey of transformation. Looking back, I would have been satisfied with just part of my recovery. Somehow, I was not to give up, there was something destined for me. Even though I was completely blind to what awaited me, onward I went.

The Monster

It was during the early years after the injury when I began referring to the pain as, "The Monster." *The Monster* started out as physical pain; back pain, muscle pain, nerve pain, and pain from the scar tissue buildup. Then *The Monster* added in mental health challenges which included anxiety, depression, medical C-PTSD, and dissociative amnesia. *The Monster* was determined to end me.

Little did I know, at the time, it was the beginning of a path which was to become very unique. Each time *The Monster* dragged me back into its darkness, I was receiving another lesson. I repeatedly walked through the deepest darkness of pain and despair one could imagine. Places no one should ever know about, much less experience. I wanted to quit many times. Flashbacks still come up; triggers from random situations still startle me.

Completely Unaccepting

Somehow, I held onto *Hope,* or perhaps *Hope* held onto me. Over time *Hope* became *Instilled* in me and became my driving force. While I had nothing to base my feelings on, I felt my life was not going to end in the darkness of pain. For many years this Hope was not a burning desire, yet it was a constant flame guiding me when I needed help.

In 2002 one doctor wrote in a report: "He is completely unaccepting of the fact that he is going to have to live with things the way they are and that there is not some magical solution around the corner." Looking back now I am glad I was completely unaccepting.

I did become stuck in wanting my life back while trying to live with the pain. Like most people, I wished for my life before everything happened. I wanted to be cured. When I tried to look for ways to recover from my chronic pain, I became overwhelmed with the vast amount of information and what seemed like countless differing opinions. What was good and what wasn't? The frustration would come so quickly and I would shut down. Everyone felt they had "The" answer, if only I paid some amount of money. When you are living with chronic pain, it becomes very difficult to sift through treatments and therapies being presented.

This was on top of being completely on my own to figure out what to do. I had no support network. That was something I felt no one should ever experience and I wished to do something to help others.

My pain and life education continued for almost three decades. While it was filled with bitter sorrow, there was a shining light at the end of my journey. The time finally came to write not only about my journey, but more importantly, to create a program for others to follow. It was time to build an action-based program for others living with chronic pain.

I traveled my path without support and encouragement. Today, I have the opportunity to reach out my hand to others. While I felt alone, others can discover they are not alone.

The purpose of this chapter is to share what brought me back from extreme darkness. It is a path, a program to follow. There are stages which each person can work on at their own pace. Life is so often out of order, my sisters and brothers living with chronic pain (including chronic illness and the accompanying mental health challenges) face so much more.

This program allows people to take back some control of their lives. Chronic pain tends to take our lives captive. From the pain, medications, therapies and surgeries, to lives disrupted, relationships damaged or lost; we often feel control has been taken away.

Pain management programs are missing one key element: peer-to-peer support. There needs to be a place not only to vent, which has value, but to begin the healing journey.

The path I blindly wandered along has been turned into path never before created; yet it has the potential to make positive changes in people's lives. There are no guarantees with this program, nor in life, just an offering of Hope.

While our pain may never go away completely, it is possible to improve the quality of our lives.

Here are the stages I traveled along the path to my healing:

> *Stage 1:* Acknowledge that pain has adversely impacted the quality of our life.

> *Stage 2:* Believe in our self. There is something inside which helped us reach this point.

> *Stage 3:* Grieve the loss of things in our lives that our pain has taken from us.

> *Stage 4:* Commit to Educate ourselves about our condition.

> *Stage 5:* Forgive ourselves and others for what has taken place because of our pain.

Stage 6: Apologized to ourselves and others for any pain caused from our situation.

Stage 7: Stay in Constant Contact with fellow pain suffers for peer support.

Stage 8: Stand Up for ourselves with service providers, self-advocate for our rights.

Stage 9: Adopt and Adapt to lifestyle changes necessary to improve our quality of life.

Stage 10: Reach Out to others after having walked through the stages ourselves.

These are the stages I walked through and are the core beliefs in our support group model. They have not only helped me to exist during my darkest days, but to survive and to live again. Everyone's pain is different, and their results will also be unique because we each are unique and amazing.

Today I have my weight under control by changing my diet. I have been off all opioid pain medications for several years. I am stronger today than I have ever been in my life despite my health challenges. Join me.

Heather Hirschman

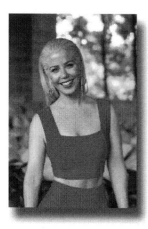

After being diagnosed with chronic Lyme disease, Heather was given an 8-year death sentence which she refused to accept.

Through her faith and perseverance, she endured, healed, and now endeavors to help clients overcome their health struggles by turning their life around.

Will you also refuse to accept your sentence?

The exciting news is once you've overcome your health struggles, you too will find your purpose, as she has found hers.

She can help you do just that.

"If you're going through hell, keep going."
~ Winston Churchill ~

Houston, Texas, USA

Website: www.purebodycoach.com

Social Media:
- www.instagram.com/yourpurebodycoach
- www.facebook.com/purebodycoach

Book a complimentary consult if you're tired of doing it alone and want answers and solutions.

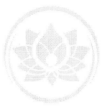

No Guts, No Glory!

The Meeting of The Brains

The hipbone is connected to the backbone... The lyrics to this well-known children's song illustrates how our body is connected, and as an adult, it is our responsibility to understand the relationship between mind and body, specifically your gut.

In order to cultivate a healthy gut and mind, we must focus on reducing and removing symptoms such as digestive distress, belly bloat, weight gain, and low energy.

Gut health impacts everything! Absolutely everything. We know that a strong gut is not just needed to digest foods and absorb nutrients, but it truly plays a profound influence on our entire body.

It's True! Your Gut Has a Brain too!

It's called the enteric nervous system. The nerve cells in our stomach, which consist of over 100 million cells, determine our overall health. The gut and the brain are two organs connected, biochemically and physically. The gut can upset the brain and vice versa.

Situational stress on the body can affect how the gut works. Bloating, weight gain, stomach aches, digestive discomfort, food allergies, sluggishness after eating, effects of medication prescribed for anxiety or depression; manifests itself in a host of undesirable ways. In the 17th century, Rene Descartes, an Italian philosopher posited that the mind and body are separate but can affect each other. A dualist relationship. If our body is talking to us through symptoms and we choose to ignore it, then it will be at our own peril.

The Good News

Imagine approaching a dark tunnel you plan to drive through. Suddenly, there are flashing lights and a sign says, "Do not enter". Do you keep driving? Heck, no.

Listen to your intuition. Maybe you have a gut feeling that something just isn't right with your body? The feeling of butterflies in your tummy? These sensations from your belly running upward to your mind, illustrate the close connection between the gut and brain. You must pay attention to this connection, or stress and being overweight will be a constant problem; or, unfortunately a chronic disease may be in your future.

If the digestive system is left unattended creating food allergies, celiac disease, and inflammation, the result may be leaky gut. The good news is, the body can repair and heal itself, with appropriate care, most significantly using food as medicine.

What's Your Body Type?

Are you trying to lose 5, 10, or 20 pounds and you've tried that diet you heard, read or been told about, where everybody lost inches and pounds? You tried it, and gained 5 pounds and felt even more sluggish. What in the world, right? Amiright? Or Amiright?

Everyone has a different body type based upon DNA & genetics. There is a reason that diets may not be working for you. It is important to determine your body type so the foods you are consuming will help you feel energetic, keep the pounds off, look your best, and keep illness away.

Overweight people resort to comfort based foods or overeat. Consumption of comfort based foods spike insulin levels, which store fat.

Did you know our gut tells us what food we want?

The other component to weight gain is that bacteria in your gut tells you what it needs to eat in order to survive. We can be so hard on ourselves when we experience uncontrollable cravings when the cravings are actually those of the bacteria and not from our lack of willpower. The answer? Eat foods that support and balance our bodies, for nourishment but that starves the bacteria residing in our gut.

Foods to Increase to support brain and gut health:

Avocado, omega 3 fats (oily fish, fermented foods (df yogurt, sauerkraut, df cheese), high fiber-foods (nuts, seeds, fruits & veggies, prebiotics, probiotics, whole grains (in moderation), olive oil, green tea, turkey, eggs.

Foods to Decrease:

Red meat, gluten, dairy, spicy and acidic foods, processed foods and sugar, caffeine, and alcohol.

Alternatives may be implemented if you happen to have food sensitivities to any of the above suggestions.

Bacterium not only controls our food cravings but also can be the reason for anxiety, depression and emotional symptoms that follow.

Relaxation is the Name of the Game

Are anxiety and depression adversely affecting your ability to control your eating (food choices and quantity)? I have found that both active and passive relaxation activities help to alleviate the manifestations of both anxiety and depression.

Active activities include massages (my favorite type is Thai), reflexology, and a variety of exercises. Passive activities include listening to music, writing in a journal, reading, drinking a warm cup of tea, meditation, immersion in art, and coloring books.

I believe we're all looking for answers to be able to achieve a happy and healthy life. If one could snap their fingers and their health comes into alignment, we would rejoice and yell it from the rooftop; however, it will take time, effort, hard work, and consistency on your part to achieve.

How Stressed Are You?

Did you know that about 95% of all illnesses are either caused or exacerbated by stress? These stressors can be chemical, physical, or emotional in origin. It is believed by an overwhelming number of doctors and professionals that the main culprit of all disease is stress.

It may surprise you to learn that the body cannot differentiate between different types of stress, positive or negative in nature. Some stress is good to allow the body to pump adrenaline and be reminded it's still alive.

Stressors cause the body to react and be out of balance as illustrated below:

1. The things that affect emotional health are finances, job, family loss, and relationships. Eastern Medicine and Energy Medicine say that as human beings, we have learned to hold on to all of our emotions or suppress them. This creates density in our bodies which western medicine has identified as a series of emotional and physical disorders with diagnoses such as cancer, fibromyalgia, anxiety, depression, and headaches. Learn to let it out, or a domino effect may occur.

2. Physical health like accidents or injuries, muscle tension and tightness

3. Chemical Stress as a result of the environment, bacteria, viruses, foods, heavy metals, hang overs, blood sugar levels

The Solution:

Stress amplifies pain, illness, and addiction to foods. We don't want to add in medications to mask the problem; rather, we must incorporate natural practices to help reduce the stress which will reduce the pain.

The goal needs to be to get to the root components of your health. Quick fixes, which include medication or what is known as "band-aid diagnoses", simply don't work long term and often times lead to serious health problems.

Are You Living in The Present?

The future remains to be seen, and the past is just that! Therefore, I believe the idea of health and wellness both in the mind and gut is only sustained when studied and practiced continuously. Not only do our bodies change, but also our environment changes day after day, year after year. Remember Hurricane Harvey in Houston, Texas in 2017 and the changes it brought?

You may only be in the present if you are aware of the current research and are making the necessary adjustments to an ever evolving and changing world. Science shows that every organ in the human body has the ability to heal itself given the proper environment, proper lifestyle and nutrition. Consequently, incorporating the above suggestions, will guide you in taking monumental steps towards restoring your body to full health. Research supports the body replaces cells about every 7-10 years. So what is one thing you will do today to contribute to a healthy mind, body, and gut? Just one! The road may be rough initially but ... No Guts, No Glory!

"It's not the stress that kills us, it is our reaction to it."
~ Hans Selye ~

Archana Amlapure

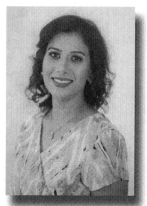

Archana Amlapure, a health coach and Yoga therapist, is on a mission to spread the knowledge about the best ways to lead a healthy, happy, and joyful life.

She believes that meditation is the most comprehensive way to achieve perfect balance between all aspects of health like physical, mental, emotional, and spiritual.

Having worked in corporate industry for 12+ years, she has an acute sense of problems the corporate lifestyle can lead to.

She has helped many individuals across all age groups and genders to achieve the true sense of mindfulness and stability.

Residing in Singapore with her husband and two kids, she pursues her passion to help as many individuals to help them find harmony, health and happiness.

"Meditation is a vital way to purify and quiet the mind.
Thus, rejuvenating the body."
~ Deepak Chopra ~

Singapore

Website: www.ojasyog.com

Social Media:
- www.facebook.com/ojasyog
- www.linkedin.com/in/archana-amlapure-ba166632/

Meditate to Revive, Rejuvenate, and Recharge Life

"**I** am feeling peaceful, pleasant, and placid," said John.

Six months ago, he approached me complaining about stress, anxiety, and lack of focus. He was distressed, dejected, and disconnected. After diagnosis, I had administered Yoga therapy for him with the focus on daily meditation. Now, I could see increased enthusiasm, productivity, comfort, and calmness on his face.

Having lived a corporate life and experienced stress and anxiety firsthand, I can attest that meditation has helped me tremendously. It has enabled me to discover my soul and my passion. I am truly grateful for being a follower of, and guide to, this ancient practice which is still pertinent today.

Whenever I ask the audience in my classes, workshops or talks, people tell me they are stressed and anxious. They always feel rushed and exhausted. Many have sleep issues and constantly deal with aches and pains.

In the modern world, where social media is an ubiquitous part of our lives, we are connected 24/7. All the information we can imagine is available at one touch. In a true sense, we are disconnecting from our self—in other words, disconnecting from our happiness. Today's lifestyle of abundance is disturbing our health and happiness.

Our whole day is rammed full of hectic commutes, endless email, high-pressure meetings, taking care of household chores and kids, and social engagements. This keeps the mind busy and agitated, constantly thinking and worrying.

It has created hazardous health problems like stress, anxiety, depression, hypertension, diabetes, back pain, obesity, migraine. These conditions are called lifestyle-related disorders. It has not only affected physical health but personal leisure time, relationships, productivity, focus and sleep, etc.

Meditation is increasing in popularity to alleviate the above problems. It is an ancient practice. In olden times, the purpose was to find enlightenment and moksha. Today, it is helping modern-age people to correct their lifestyle and find solace. It's not simply a buzzword; rather, it is supported by scientific proof. Many psychologists and neurologists are studying the benefits of meditation.

What is Meditation?

Meditation is the process of being aware of what is going on within you and around you. It is about focusing and turning one's senses inwards. Meditation is simply focusing on the present moment.

Different tools like breathing, sounds or objects are used during meditation. But the purpose is the same: to reduce unnecessary traffic of thoughts and simply focus on the breath or a single thought.

Scientific Study

Modern scientific instruments and techniques like MRI and ECG have shown the changes in the brain that result from meditation. A research study [1] shows that meditation increases the density of grey matter, which thickens the prefrontal cortex. This helps in refining executive functions of the prefrontal cortex like the ability to differentiate among conflicting thoughts, determine good and bad, identify future consequences of current activities, working toward a defined goal.

Another study showed meditation helps to reduce the beta level of mind [2]. Meaning, meditation reduces the number of thoughts, bringing clarity and making one a better decision-maker.

Meditation also reduces the fight-or-flight response by reducing stress hormones such as cortisol, which leads to making better decisions at times of crisis. It makes one a better leader.

In addition, meditation has shown the benefits of reducing chronic stress and anxiety, improving concentration, enhancing self-awareness, increasing productivity, and improving immunity response.

From my experience of working with people with these conditions, meditation has helped them to bring harmony in their thoughts, put a conscious mind to rest, and slow down. This helps them to manage their stress, relationships, and health. Now, they enjoy pain-free lives. Meditation has become an integral part of their daily routine.

It is said that true happiness cannot be found outside, but lies within. Meditation is an effective way to go inwards.

Myths About Meditation

Though it sounds simple, many people find it difficult to meditate. Indeed, many are still skeptical about meditation. They believe they can't concentrate, sit still, or control their thoughts. Still others associate meditation with religious practice.

"Meditation is not concentration. Concentration is a result of meditation."

Meditation requires patience, self-discipline, and consistency. It will seem like a time-consuming activity until you start experiencing the benefits of it. These will only be availed with discipline and patience.

Meditation is a New Medication

Meditation is acting like a new medication for these modern diseases. For example, when we seek help for migraines, only painkillers are prescribed. These painkillers work on symptoms such as headache. But the root cause of the headaches might be stress, anxiety, or hormonal changes. So, what is the root cause? The mind. Research shows that one in four people in the world will be affected by a mental disorder. [3]

To heal the mind, the best medicine is meditation.

Meditation acts as antibiotics rather than painkillers. Many people have found relief from their busy mind and health problems with this powerful medicine.

Meditation is for Everyone

The best part of meditation is, it is for everyone. For those who are healthy, it is like health insurance, and for those who are suffering from diseases, it is like a medicine. It is equally effective for kids and teens to build self-esteem and improve focus in studies and memory.

Meditation as a Winning Strategy

Nowadays, awareness of meditation is on the rise. Even corporations are realizing the importance of meditation for improving employee health, engagement, and productivity. More and more executives are embracing this practice to become successful leaders.

Many employers are investing in creating mental health by adapting meditation techniques in their work environment.

People who have good health, have strong control over emotions, and have achieved success regularly meditate. A lot of successful people have used meditation as a strategy for winning and being successful.

How to Build a Sustainable Meditation Routine:

1. Consistency and self-discipline are important for better results

2. Choose what suits you: There are many methods available for meditation, such as breath, sound, transcendental, dynamic meditation, and more. Choose what suits you best. Best is to learn from an expert teacher/practitioner.

3. Allot a fixed time: Prioritize and allocate a fixed time during the day and meditate at the same time. Mediation can be done anytime during the day, but sunrise and sunset is best, when all of nature is meditating. You can easily focus on the breath and experience peace.

4. Choose the right place: Try to meditate in the same place every day. It can be a corner of your room or at your office cubicle. It helps to create an aura and positive vibrations.

5. No prejudice: Try not to be judgmental about your experiences. Don't judge the outcome or the feelings that arise during meditation. Sometimes emotions come to the surface during meditation, but they will eventually dissolve.

6. Be patient: Initially, you may simply feel nothing helps, but keep going. Patience will lead to consistent practice and sustained results.

7. Consistency: Meditation is not a one-time job, but rather needs to be done repeatedly to enjoy the benefits.

8. Breath meditation: The best and simplest meditation technique is to focus on the breath, either the tip of your nose or the rise of the chest or belly with inhaling and exhaling. Anytime the mind wanders, bring your attention back to breathing.

Make a promise to yourself today to make meditation part of your daily routine for a beautiful, happy, and joyous life.

When you take control of your life, life will stop taking control of you. With full authority and control, you can revive, rejuvenate and recharge every aspect of your life.

Kathleen Mulligan

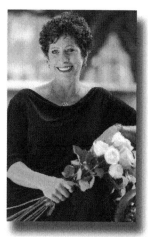

Since 2005, Kathleen Mulligan's professional dedication has been calling women to become stronger, healthier, and more resilient leaders.

Her 'whole woman' approach supports women living into their highest potential with a deepened sense of fulfillment and success – and without sacrificing the quality of their lives.

Kathleen offers her clients state of the art, best-in-class tools in Social & Emotional Intelligence, Resilience and Stress Management, Executive Presence, Well-Being, and more.

Her one-on-one and intimate group VIP retreat intensives are life-changing experiences. Kathleen is a certified Solution-Focused Transformational Coach and Leadership Consultant working with Executive and Entrepreneurial women.

"Life isn't about finding yourself. Life is about creating yourself."
~ George Bernard Shaw~

San Francisco Bay Area

Website: www.KathleenMulligan.com

Social Media:
- www.linkedin.com/in/kathleenmulligannewwaveleadership
- www.facebook.com/Kathleen-Mulligan

Want to take a powerful scientifically validated Stress and Well-Being Assessment online – and for free? "Subject: STRESSED" Kathleen@KathleenMulligan.com

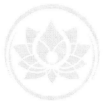

The Superpower of Pause:
In Life & Leadership

We are living in times of chaos and disruption. It's noisy out there. Most of us appear to be in a personal foot race with the speed of light itself. We are all running too fast.

In leadership circles, there's a buzz word and acronym that reflects the sign of our times. Meet VUCA. Originally coined by the US military, the term is now widely used to describe the nature of what today's leaders 'must' be able to handle to stay at the top.

VUCA, as a catch-all term, suggests, "It's insane in here!" The actual acronym stands for Volatility, Uncertainty, Complexity & Ambiguity.

I say VUCA pretty much sums up the state of affairs that each of us is facing – every single day.

What is at the heart of VUCA?

It is the ever-rising and unrelenting tide of global change that is washing over all of us at an unprecedented rate. This relentless wave of change is saturating every area of our personal and professional lives. The technology that has positively advanced our global civilization in innumerable ways has also created a type of unnatural 24/7connectivity. This extended connectivity, paradoxically, has left many of us feeling overwhelmed, disconnected from ourselves, one another, and our sense of well-being.

And so, what do VUCA, The Power of Pause and Leadership have to do with you? A lot!

I'm going to offer you a multifold answer:

Part One: Leadership

Do you believe, as I do, that there has never been a time, in our lifetime, when a new paradigm of leadership is more critically needed? If so, then "leadership" is important to you.

I believe that to grow as an effective and inspiring leader, one must learn to lead themselves first; this is Self-Leadership.

I believe every one of us has a powerful leader within.

I believe that to create sustainable change our world is desperately calling for, we must boldly call forth the leaders that live within us.

Each of us may show up as a leader in a different arena. We may lead from within our families and homes, our communities, schools, businesses, organizations, or all of the above.

When I use the term leader, I am pointing to you. Are you a person who aspires to inspire, who desires to make an impact, who can envision how to create a better future, and who will walk others towards that future? You are a leader.

I call the collective that we form through our mutual commitment to a better future, *New Wave Leadership*™. It's about you, and me, calling forth the leader within and choosing to model a way to walk towards a tomorrow that will be better than today.

Are you with me?

As a professional life and leadership development coach and consultant for over fourteen years, I am fiercely passionate about supporting women to become models for this new wave of leadership.

I believe it's time for women to take our seat at the table. I believe it's time to extend our hands filled to overflowing with our intelligence, our high-level competencies, and our inherent skills as empathetic collaborators. We will extend our hands with our intention to bridge the gap between the old way of leadership and the New Wave. The gap is wide, and we have our work cut out for us.

Remember, as leaders, we must learn to lead ourselves first. We are going to be required to step through the minefields and daily deluge of the chaos, complexity, and distractions of our ever-changing world.

Knowing this, I offer up the Power of Pause as an often-overlooked Superpower.

Part Two: The Power of Pause

The Power of Pause is a learnable skill set and practice. Like most practices, such as yoga or exercise, it can yield significant returns for our overall well-being. The concept of the Power of Pause is backed by both cutting-edge neuroscience and the ancient wisdom traditions gathered over 1000s of years.

By calling us to practice the Power of Pause, I am encouraging each of us to slow down, step back, and catch our breath. The Power of Pause is about living more consciously and intentionally.

The Power of Pause is about creating moments of rest and recovery (superior athletes know this to be crucial for sustainable high-performance). It's about creating white space wherein we can create, innovate, and explore possibilities within and outside of ourselves. When we are in chaos and stress our cortical function (the thinking/processing part of our brain) is inhibited; we do not think as clearly.

The Practice of Pause allows us to access our higher-level thinking, creativity, and decision making.

From the beginning of man's time, the pause has been an intrinsic act that has been essential to our well-being. Today, too many of us have forgotten how to make time in our lives for this creative and rejuvenating lifeforce.

As Kevin Cashman, CEO and Executive Development at Korn Ferry International, shares in his acclaimed book, *The Pause Principals*, "Pause, is the natural capability to slow down and step back in order to move forward with greater clarity, momentum, and impact…"

As a daily practice, the Power of Pause impacts our biochemical and psychophysiological states. It has the same natural transformative benefits as sleep and eating nourishing whole foods. (Has anyone noticed that both sleep and mindful nutrition seem to be slipping to the back burner or outright ignored as well?)

In our compulsively connected, achieve-more-now-crush-it world, we are progressively disconnecting from our primary human essential rhythms. It's time to commit to the Power and Practice of Pause.

Final Part: Tying it all together

We are living in times of chaos and disruption... We are all running too fast.

To begin cultivating your unique Power of Pause practice allow me to suggest three very simple prompts. (do not let their simplicity fool you):

1. *Pause:*
   Before you do anything. Before you pick up the phone, enter the room, before you speak, before you decide to say 'yes' or 'no,' before you push send — Pause. Get in the habit of pausing and being present to who you are being in that moment. What actions are you intentionally taking? Be conscious of the outcome you intend to create.

2. *Pause and Breathe:*
   Nothing can reset our natural rhythms more quickly or efficiently than taking a few slow, deep breaths into our heart and belly area. If you can also generate a feeling of appreciation and gratitude as you slowly breathe in and out of your heart area, you will shift your entire bio, and psychophysiological chemistry as you do. You'll access higher cortical function, increase your energy, and bring a more optimal state of being, in an instant.

3. *Pause with a Purpose:*
   Set a quiet alarm randomly throughout your day. When the alarm sounds, run through a quick series of questions:

   - Who am I being in this situation?
   - What is important in this moment?
   - How can I contribute to making this moment more meaningful, for myself and others?

So often we move through our days on auto-pilot. Use the Power of Pause to begin living more intentionally and on purpose.

To build bridges to a better tomorrow, we need a new wave of leaders today. Overwhelmed, wired-up, and burned-out people are not going to get us there. We need you. We need inspiring, focused, and energized leaders who have a deepened sense of self-awareness and a commitment to a brighter future. That self-awareness can only be found within the quiet space of the pause.

I invite you to join me there and begin practicing the Power of Pause today.

"Live life as though everything is rigged in your favor."
~ Rumi ~

Dr. Karen Stillman

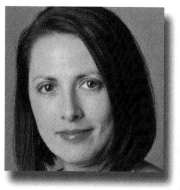

Dr. Karen Stillman is a retired Obstetrician/ Gynecologist turned Transformation Life Coach.

She primarily serves women in their wellness domain.

After twelve years of a heart centered practice and having her own health challenges, she found she and her clients are best served by using evocative coaching principles and *The Spiritual Laws of Success.*

This is science at its' fullest, expressing energy in the most positive ways for amazing results.

Karen resides in Ottawa, ON, Canada, where she serves clients around the globe.

"Imagination is more important than knowledge."
~ Albert Einstein ~

Ottawa, Ontario, Canada

Website: www.karenstillman.dreambuildercoach.com/

Social Media:
- www.facebook.com/sacredspacewithkaren
- www.linkedin.com/in/karen-stillman-7078b410/
- www.instagram.com/sacredspacewithkaren/

Enhance your fertility. Become pregnant. Have a baby. Contact me for a proven and reliable system. sacredspacewithkaren@gmail.com; 613-314-9802

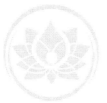

Your Abundant Uterus:
Thinking Into Pregnancy

"We cannot solve our problems with the same thinking
we used when we created them."
~ Albert Einstein ~

You want to have a baby. You are not where you wanted to be. However, you find yourself reading this chapter because you are ready for a change in your results. This chapter is written to help you break free from your current challenges with fertility, reconnect you with the infinite side of your BE-ing, and awaken the hidden power within you to transform your life to create the baby you desire.

I'm going to share with you a framework to start a process of changing your thoughts to enhance your fertility and create the family you would love.

There is a mountain of information in the medical field about diagnosis, testing, and treating a suitcase full of complaints. I know. I have tested, prescribed and done thousands of procedures. With all the medical information available today, and you have probably used some of it, are you having the results you wanted? No? Western Medicine typically does not follow the Spiritual Laws of Universal Success. It is looking to change conditions by doing things to you. Telling you how you are. This is external. Up until now, you may have let it.

The true cause of a successful pregnancy and spontaneous vaginal childbirth is within you. You have the power. Take it back! Yes, you may make use of medical services and tools for your success. That is okay. They are part of the Universe's resources.

For every problem, there already exists a solution [1]. The Universe is abundant with resources for you. Your uterus is like the Universe. It is mostly empty space ready to be filled with and grow your baby.

You are a perfect spiritual being having a human experience [2]. Everything you need is available to you. Your mind has the power to unlock the code.

It is done by accessing your six mental faculties.

Your six mental faculties are Imagination, Intuition, Will, Memory, Reason, and Perception. They are wonderful gifts which allow you to move beyond your current circumstances, situations, and conditions. We all have these gifts. Our different results are based on how we use, or misuse them.

"You can't get to your dream, you must come from it. [3]" You can have anything you are willing to become. What is your greatest desire?

I will describe each faculty as they are taught in Bob Proctor and Mary Morrissey's *Into Your Genius*™ program. The seven steps that follow is my outline to help you start a process of enhancing your fertility and creating the baby and family you would love.

Imagination

The first step begins with the end. By using your imagination and knowing what you would love is key to be holding your baby. Everything you see around you was first a thought before it became a thing. Your thoughts are the most powerful energy there is! [4]

Dream up what it is you desire. Start by asking yourself this question: "What would I love?" See yourself in this dream life three years from now. What does it look like? Write it down. Be as specific as you can. Include descriptions that use all of your five senses. How many children do you have? What does your typical day look like? What do you feel when you hold your baby? How does he/she smell?

Allow yourself to lean in, feeling the love. This is your life! It is your dream come true. You only need to know the 'what' right now. Put the 'how' on hold. Notice how your body responds to this movie of you holding your baby.

Michael Beckwith says, "Energy flows where your attention goes." Believe in your dream. Trust this process.

Intuition

The next step involves using your intuition to receive answers from the Universe or Infinite Intelligence. There is not a question you can ask that doesn't already have an answer. [5] This knowing is available when you listen, in the calm and quiet.

How well do you listen? Do you follow the answers?

Or are you logically or rationally making assumptions based on facts and circumstances rather than truths?

Your mind is connected to all the minds in the Universe. [6] This knowing is often called your still small voice. It comes as hunches, nudges and gut feelings. You are powerful as you are truly connected.

The Will

You have the image of the life you would love with baby. You are listening to your still small voice for the next step. Your Will allows you to focus and concentrate on your dream of a baby and lets the resources you need flow to you.

This is not "will power". If the force of will power worked, most all the New Years' Resolutions would be achieved! There is no force or struggle here.

Continuous and sustained mental thought is one of the biggest challenges people face today. [7] Most shy away from it, looking to the facts outside (a diagnosis) rather than the truth. The truth is you have the ability to create what you want to create, including your health, and a baby.

Do not set out contingency plans or other options. Clear mental focus on being pregnant and holding your baby is essential. Continuous calm thoughts allow the resources you need to come to you. Remember that "energy flows where your attention goes".

Memory

Your memory is perfect. Not only is it perfect, it works backwards and forwards! Most of us are lead to believe we have a poor memory. Do you practice and work with your memory? Like athletes working to become the next Olympian, they practice. It takes time and practice to be aware and sense Infinite Intelligence.

Did you know your mind cannot tell the difference between a past or future event? When you keep telling your mind you are pregnant, it works to maintain that image. The flow of information and resources to assist you with this is astounding! It's like going back to the future. You come from the dream.

Your body will work towards this because in your mind, it is already done. You told it so. Your future self, holding your baby, has information for you to use right now. Ask yourself what it is. It will open doors and make things easier.

As you hold the image of being pregnant in your mind, you are in a vibrational match with this result. Feel this positive energy. Make it yours today.

Reason

The information from your five senses is a representation of your current state of reality: your current results. This is a reflected reality of what you are thinking. [8]

It is the facts of your history with your permission – you have infertility or recurrent pregnancy loss. You cannot make or have a baby.

Your reasoning faculty allows you to think through each situation you are facing. Forcing or pushing energy often does not allow us to have the success we desire. When you allow and make welcome what it is you desire, the solution becomes available. It's like a map to get you where you want to be.

Use right reasoning to remember you have perfect imagination, intuition, and memory. [9] Recognize you are connected to the best "Internet" there is: Infinite Intelligence. You are increasing your sense of deserving. Bring a willingness to make the baby you desire welcome. Tune into this vibration. Turn away from the "problems". Follow the right map.

Perception

How do you interpret your surroundings? Only you have the power to make yourself think a thought. No one else can make you feel a certain way without your permission.

Every situation is neutral. You assign it bad or good. There will always be challenges. Know that everything is good. There is a lesson or gift in every situation. You may not know the exact meaning or purpose of how it is good at the present moment. This is okay. Hold a place for the gift. Revisit the lesson later.

Press an "internal pause button" [10] on any situation where your initial reaction is "that's bad!" Plan to react three days later – no sooner. Then look at it from a different point of view. Fear may have been an enemy. Let it walk with you as your friendly reminder that you're on the growing edge to success. Remain calm and let the Universe know you are open to an idea. This is where practicing forgiveness and gratitude will change your results.

Forgiveness is a shift in your perception which removes a block within you, to your awareness of love in any situation. [11] That love may be more or less skillfully delivered. Holding onto anger or resentment in any aspect of your life only holds you back from your highest good. This includes getting pregnant and having a baby. This is hard work. It will not change the past. It will change who you are today and transform your future.

Gratitude is a practice of being thankful for everything and in every situation that comes your way. Gratitude is on the same vibrational frequency as love. A gratitude practice increases the flow of goodness into your life.

Summary

You are the architect of your life. Don't live by default as a victim of conditions and circumstances. Design and build your dream. Get pregnant. Have a baby. Live the life you would love with the family you desire.

This outline I designed of the seven steps to enhancing your fertility is merely the beginning. Enjoy!

1. Write out your dream in detail. Start with "I am so happy and grateful now that". Read it twice daily. Feel the positive energy.

2. Make time for quiet reflection. Remain focused. Welcome information as it flows to you.

3. Practice gratitude daily for everything in your life, including the pregnant Moms and babies you see. Know that is you as well. Keep a gratitude journal with your lists.

4. Practice forgiveness. Release yourself and others unto their highest good.

5. Turn failures into feedback. Remove any emotional charge from them. Ask "what is the lesson here"?

6. Try writing a letter to the part(s) of your body which are challenging you. What does it say to you?

7. Ask daily "What can I do today to move me in the direction of my dream?"

Know that you are perfection. You can have whatever you desire, choose and are willing to become. Trust in the Universe. Believe in your uterus. The power to become pregnant and have a baby is within you!

Ursula Wood

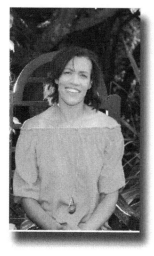

Ursula Wood is an accredited trainer and performance coach who specialises in providing personal resilience coaching and training.

She's also a wellbeing devotee who believes wellness is unique and there is no one-shoe-fits-all when it comes to managing or improving it.

Her strong desire for others to seek wellness solutions that best suit them led her to become the co-founder of *Wellbeing Umbrella*, where she is committed to working with other wellness practitioners to help her achieve the ultimate goal – connecting people to a world full of options for the purpose of enhancing individual and workplace wellness.

"Life is simple. Everything happens for you, not to you.
Everything happens at exactly the right moment, neither too soon nor too late.
You don't have to like it… it's just easier if you do."
~ Byron Katie ~

Bradford, West Yorkshire, United Kingdom

Website: www.wellbeingumbrella.com

Social Media:
- www.facebook.com/wellbeingumbrella
- www.instagram.com/wellbeingumbrella
- www.facebook.com/wellbeingumbrellabusiness

Score & improve your resilience with our FREE questionnaire, eBook download, and monthly wisdom. http://bit.ly/WellbeingUmbrellaResilienceResource

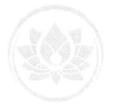

3 Steps to Improve Your Resilience

Have you ever noticed how some people are seemingly fortunate not to be fazed by significant pressures, while others (the large majority of us) wilt under what seems a minor stress? This doesn't mean we are less able or capable of coping, it just means we need to develop and strengthen our everyday resilience a little further.

What is Resilience?

Everyday resilience is what gives you the ability to stay strong and recover quickly from anything life throws at you; including life's setbacks or daily challenges. You know, those unexpected repair bills, a relationship break up, the relentless commute to work, that project that didn't quite go as planned, or that one toxic person who's never happy with you no matter what.

Everyday resilience enables you to adapt and grow, so that the way you view and tackle your outer world has a lesser impact upon you. There are 5 key areas that make up your everyday resilience:

1. Mindset
Having, or developing, a positive and flexible mentality which enables you to approach challenges with an optimistic attitude while remaining confident and motivated.

2. Empowerment
Believing in yourself and your ability to do well.

3. Moral Compass
Being aware of what is important to you and knowing the direction of which you wish to take in life.

4. Emotional Choice

Being able to manage and negotiate how you want to emotionally respond to situations and people.

5. Supportive Circles

Looking after your own needs first before giving to others (healthy selfishness); being aware of your own limitations and getting support to meet.

Being aware of your limitations and continually developing within any of the five areas of everyday resilience is what can make the difference between a slight wobble and being completely flawed when faced with life's challenges or setbacks.

For the purpose of this chapter, I will concentrate on the second key area of resilience; 'empowerment' and explore some practical ways to help you manage self-doubt!

The art of managing self-doubt is recognising how it occurs. When we experience self-doubt, it is essentially our emotions giving us a warning that our safety or happiness could be at threat (survival instinct). This warning system drives us to take action so that we can feel safe again; the only problem is the rational part of the brain tends to no longer get a look in.

A great example of this occurring is when someone is offered an opportunity to speak in public, yet unhelpful thoughts about their ability begin to manifest. Their internal voice taunts and criticises them, making them feel uncertain and uncomfortable about the opportunity. So much so they may feel driven to put an end to the emotional discomfort by declining the offer.

To manage self-doubt, you need to take active steps to strengthen the rational (decision-making) part of the brain and quieten the emotional part (survival instinct). Here are three helpful steps:

1. Finish Point

Get clear on what it is you want and write it down. Writing down what you want to accomplish naturally helps you to focus your thoughts. It's also concrete evidence of what you want, the reason you want it, and helps you to work out a plan of how you're going to achieve it.

2. Find the Pleasure

Equilibrium is the key to our survival and it's human nature for us to avoid discomfort and gravitate towards pleasure. Before we make a decision, our brain quickly works through a process of 'discomfort or pleasure' to determine which course of action is best for us, based on the least discomfort. To help you overcome the unease experienced when self-doubt raises its head, you'll need to identify 'what it will cost you' and 'what you'll gain' if you want to move out of your comfort zone.

To achieve this, write the headings 'Pleasure' and 'Cost' down on paper.

Under the heading 'Pleasure', write down all that you'll gain if you choose to address self-doubt. Ask yourself some probing questions such as: what will you gain if you decide to overcome your self-doubt/achieve your goal? How will life be different? How will you and others benefit (emotionally, physically, mindfully, and financially)? How will you talk to and treat yourself?

Now, under the heading of 'Cost', write down what it will cost you if you choose not to address your self-doubt. Ask yourself further probing questions such as: what's your self-doubt costing you and others (emotionally, physically, mindfully, and financially)? What are you missing out on? What has your self-doubt cost you in the past? How is your self-doubt affecting how you speak to/treat yourself?

3. Challenge and Replace

The next step is managing any negative or undermining thoughts and emotions which are sent as alarm signals by the brain in an attempt to protect you from moving out of your comfort zone.

The aim is to challenge any self-doubt thoughts you may have by asking yourself some more probing questions to determine whether your thoughts are true or false. The technique also supports you to look for more balanced, realistic, and beneficial ways to resolve your self-doubt and take action. Here's how:

- In a situation when you next experience feelings of self-doubt, write down the situation that triggered you to feel or react as you did. Stick to facts, no opinion or judgement is required.

- *Your emotions:* write down how the situation made you 'feel' or is currently making you feel. Also add information on how you reacted/behaved.

- *Current thinking:* write down current and/or the thoughts that led you to feel and respond as you did. Ask yourself questions such as: what's making me feel this way? What is it that I think might happen? What's really bothering me?

- *Challenge self-doubt thinking:* now you get to play judge and jury with your current thinking. Take the time to look back at what you wrote under the heading 'current thinking' as it's time to examine what evidence you have to prove whether your self-doubt statements are correct, or just unhelpful thinking that is causing you to feel bad about yourself.

Coaching Based Questions

To help you challenge the accuracy of your 'current thinking' statements, jot down your answers to them:

1. Do you have any evidence or facts to back up what you think/believe, or do you just 'think' it is true?

2. Are your feelings getting in the way of your judgement or is it based upon facts?

3. If it's true, is it always the case or just sometimes?

4. What advice would you give a good friend if they had this same thought/belief?

5. What evidence can you replace that would be a fairer take on the thought you currently have?

6. How likely is it to happen?

7. Are you 100% certain it will occur, or is it just a possibility?

8. What is the worst that could happen? And how can you best handle that?

9. What would you like to be true about 'you' in this current situation? What can you do to achieve that?

10. How important will this be to you in 1 week, 1 month or 1 year?

Final words

Remember, the journey to becoming resilient and overcoming self-doubt doesn't tend to happen overnight, so be patient with yourself and reach out to a qualified practitioner where needed.

"Life doesn't get easier or more forgiving, we get stronger and more resilient."
~ Steve Maraboli ~

Patti Beres

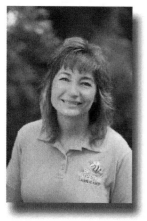

Founder and CEO of *Be Green Pro LLC.* since 2010 to provide a healthier, more responsible choice and service for people seeking lawn, insect, pest and tree care that's safer for people, pets, properties, and the planet.

First and always a believer, woman, wife, mother, daughter, sister, friend, learner and teacher.

Born a free spirit who holds a magical passion for all things "nature".

Thus far, spending a lifetime advocating for environmental sustainability coexisting with human stewardship on behalf of the planet and all creatures we have been gifted.

Thirty plus years of knowledge and "green" industry experience from family business, formal education, learning from horticultural experts and ongoing on-the-job training.

Mission: Create awareness and provide choices that empower people to reduce the chemical footprint in their lives and communities.

"If you change the way you look at things, the things you look at change."
~ Wayne Dyer ~

Oconomowoc, Wisconsin, USA

Website: www.begreen.pro

Social Media:
- www.facebook.com/begreenpro/
- www.twitter.com/Begreenlawn
- www.linkedin.com/in/patriciaberes/

Servicing Southeastern WI - contact us today for a fee estimate
https://begreen.pro/contact/

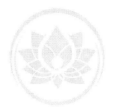

Five Tips for Growing Your Best Lawn
- Naturally -

Do you love your lawn? If so, you are in good company with millions of American homeowners, and rightfully so!

Grassy lawn areas provide a velvety green carpet of luxurious beauty and comfort which surrounds your home and your most valuable asset, your family.

A well kept lawn provides a monetary increase in home value, as well as, measurable health benefits such as oxygen, air quality, temperature moderation, sound insulation, water filtration, erosion control, and natural habitat for beneficial natural wildlife.

The last 40 years has witnessed a dramatic change in lawn care practices and use of toxic chemicals. Homeowners make decisions to trust products and professionals in the best interest of providing picturesque, golf course style perfection for their home and family, often at a chemically toxic cost.

Here are my five favorite tips for growing your best lawn - naturally:

1. Nutrition

We all need the best food possible to keep fit and healthy. Your lawn is no different. Fertilizer is supplemental nutrition, or lawn food. Just like food in your local market, not all are created the same and there are so many choices! Labels are tricky to read and its important to understand content and application instructions.

What's actually in those packages? Many are synthetic nitrogen based and contain more cheap fillers than nutrients! Likewise, hiring a professional should include research of their products, practices, and values.

Giving your lawn an all-natural, compost or organic based slow-release product provides long lasting feeding that encourages living soil (beneficial soil microbes) which promote deep roots and produces thick green growth.

Doing this makes it naturally more resistant to weeds, disease, insects and drought. I recommend application every 6 - 8 weeks.

This is not an area to compromise, but if budget requires you must, spring and fall are the most important. Fall is when your lawn is absorbing all the nutrition it needs to go to sleep for the winter. Just like animals hibernate, your lawn does too. Your lawn doesn't die in the winter; it's sleeping and needs nutrition for vibrant spring awakening. Similar to bears coming out of their dens very thin after their long winter's nap, your spring lawn has used up all of it's stored nutrition. It is starving to be fed again. Additional feedings in early summer through fall reduce stress when grasses need additional strength in order to thrive and overcome harsh weather conditions.

2. Mowing Your Lawn

Many people envision achieving a manicured golf course style lawn as their picture of perfection. It's important to remember that golf courses hire full-time caretakers to provide continuous daily care for mowing, fertilizing, aerating, and prevention of weeds, insects, and disease. Unless you have a full-time caretaker, mowing your lawn as short as a golf course is just not a great idea.

The best practice is to cut high about once per week. Shorter mowing can scalp lawns; a sure way to thinning, bare spots that are easy targets for weeds, disease, and insects.

Food and water are stored in the tips of grass blades. When you mow, the root system actually has to work harder to seek nutrients that replenish the loss. Grass that is too long or too short causes root exhaustion from nutrient delivery which promotes overall decline. By cutting only a small portion off the top, you are allowing needed energy to remain in the roots. For a thick lawn you'll love to look at and walk on, set mower deck between 3-4" high during the summer months. Leave clippings on the lawn as long as they are not in "haystacks" which smother and cause bare spots.

Lower deck height to 2" for the last fall cutting when your lawn is ready to sleep and uses less energy. This will help deter damage from freezing and thawing, snow mold, and critters such as moles and voles who dig and tunnel. Lastly, sharpen mower blades at least once per year for a clean cut. Dull mower blades produce brown tips, torn grass blades, and diseased lawns. If you hire a professional mowing crew, discuss whether their policies and procedures align with your values.

3. Watering

You can't control nature. Weather conditions are ever-changing. Some seasons are really rainy and others are extremely dry. A healthy lawn with deeper roots is naturally more drought resistant, but when dryness lingers too long, it's appropriate to water your lawn about 1" per week if your community allows it.

Avoid watering during midday heat when evaporation or burning can cause damage, and evening hours when mold and mildew can grow. Irrigation can be your lawns best friend when used properly and sparingly.

Excessive moisture from rain or over-watering can cause problems too. Symptoms range from yellowing or discoloration, to fungus and disease. Consult a professional when choosing a lawn seed variety that will grow best in your geographic area and pay close attention to soil type, drainage, typical moisture levels, proximity to mature trees, and sunlight conditions which can all factor into moisture levels.

4. Aeration and Overseeding

Understanding aeration was a journey for me. In a perfect world, if you're following the right steps to maintain a naturally based lawn, there is a cycle of conditions, including beneficial microbes, which compost thatch and create aeration naturally. However, this ideal synergy is prohibited by changes in environmental conditions created by building foundational structures, roadways, subdivisions, homes, and changing landscapes combined with foot traffic, freezing, and thawing.

Your lawn is grown to use and enjoy. It's a place you should love to spend time without worry. It is the most magnificent place to relax, regenerate your soul and spirit, grow relationships with family, friends and pets, and play!. Investing in aeration, with or without overseeding, decompacts soil to recreate ideal lawn growing conditions.

The aeration process uses equipment that pulls a small soil core out of the ground. The holes and cores erode loosely back into place. Loose soil improves absorption of nutrition, water and air, and gives the roots room to stretch. Overseeding introduces new varieties of grass seed cultivars that strengthen disease resistance, encourage thick growth, improve general health and beauty, and produces rich even color tones.

5. Embrace Diversity

This sounds easy but is often practiced with resistance until you learn to love it! Americans have become conditioned to believe that anything other than grass is an intolerable blemish. Embracing diversity in nature is as important as embracing the diversity of our fellow human beings.

All planetary living species rely on other species in some way for survival. Certain species thrive best under special conditions while other species can't survive at all without a specific species. People have the ability to form opinions and take action regarding what species are important or annoying, and some are just unknowingly misunderstood.

For example, a "weed" is defined as something that grows where you didn't plant it, or don't want it. Dandelions and moss are two common causes of complaint. Yet, certain countries actually cultivate dandelions for their edible leaves which are higher in nutrient content than any other salad green, and use its other 'parts' for natural health remedies. Additionally, pollinators thrive where dandelions are abundant.

Moss grows especially well in shady, damp areas and can provide a lush, hardy ground cover that is soft to walk on, especially in areas where other plants struggle. Exploring new concepts in moderation can provide enjoyable simplicity where you least expect it.

The main thing to remember is that a beautiful lawn is naturally possible, available and healthier, but not necessarily perfect. Define beauty and perfection based on your values and expectations, not how someone else defines them for you.

*"And, when you want something,
all the universe conspires in helping you to achieve it."*
~ Paulo Coelho ~

Aprilani McIlwraith

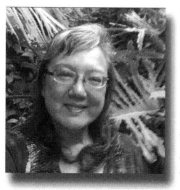

When it comes to relationships, Aprilani has read it all.

Growing up in a divorced family, Aprilani vowed not to repeat her parents' mistakes.

But with arranged marriages for role models in the rapidly changing social environment of 1960's America, she yearned for guidance to create a dream relationship.

She discovered personal development, Eastern meditation and Social Psychology but they gave only a part of the solution.

Fast forward to modern life coaching: Tony Robbins, Neuro Linguistic Programming, Hawaiian psychology, updated research, and numerous self-help books and programs later, Aprilani found that research + coaching + deep self-work to be the answer to relationship happiness.

Love yourself to build the foundation for the love of your dreams.

"Good relationships keep us happier and healthier."
~ Robert Waldinger, M.D. ~

Waipahu, Hawaii, USA

Website: www.aprilani.com

Social Media:
• www.facebook.com/AlohaAprilani/

Visit www.aprilani.com for proven ways to turn your dreams of love into the love of your dreams.

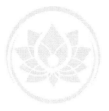

Enhance Your Wellbeing
With the Magic of Relationships

Everyone has a thought or two about their relationships. What is magical about them? How can they enhance our wellbeing?

"Good relationships keep us happier and healthier." That's according to psychiatrist Robert Waldinger, the current director of the longest study on wellbeing which is still ongoing at Harvard University. Participants in the 80 year old study who felt more satisfaction in their marriages also stayed healthier longer. The study found that "people who are more socially connected to family, to friends, to community, are happier, they're physically healthier, and they live longer than people who are less well connected" [1].

People can not only live longer, but if their relationships are strong, they are twice as likely to live longer than people with weak ties [2].

What about quality of life? Relationships can improve the quality of your life, too. There are several studies that look at different aspects. One example is that your memory can stay sharper longer if you feel you can depend on your partner when you need them [3].

Does the Quality of Your Relationships Affect Your Health and Longevity?

Okay, so being in a relationship helps us live longer. Does it really matter if the relationship is happy or not? Couples who had happier marriages over many years of surveying, also said their health was better than unhappy couples [4].

Researchers also found happy marriages are more likely to actually lengthen life spans compared to unhappy marriages [5].

And, it gets more interesting. People with the happiest relationships in middle age had the best health in their older years [6].

Sum it up by saying a good and satisfying relationship can protect your health. And it was also found that decreasing relationship dissatisfaction can add to your years [7].

How Do You Have a Great Relationship?

Closeness in marriage along with commitment for unmarried couples can provide a supportive framework for the couple. This support allows the couple to identify with and feel satisfaction [8].

Leading relationship researcher Dr. John Gottman found in over 40 years of studying thousands of couples in his university research labs, that staying connected and managing disagreements is key [9].

His four-part method is:

1. Maintain calmness
2. Speak and listen nondefensively
3. Validate your partner
4. Practice to make these techniques second nature

A follow up study of Dr. Gottman's couple therapy method, found that his techniques led to greater marital satisfaction [10]. One example of his techniques is moving towards each other instead of away from each other. Techniques like this improve a couple's closeness and joy, helping them to have happier interactions and feel better about each other and their relationship. The method also helps couples participate in and share their partner's life experience which strengthens their attachment and well-being.

Commitment in relationship goes deeper than vows taken in a ceremony. It involves consistently choosing to put the relationship on a high priority. Supporting partners in times of need and managing conflicts results in the best relationships[11].

Love Yourself as a Foundation For Self and Relationship Wellbeing

What is meant by "loving yourself?" Loving yourself means feeling peace and ease within yourself. This inner peace involves a caring way of being with yourself. There is no judgment or negativity, there's kindness and acceptance.

Does loving yourself really improve your love relationship? Although long-time therapists have found this with their patients, researchers are in the process of exploring these links. They are far from finding conclusive evidence to say one causes the other. Relationships, love and human behavior in general are complicated, defined in different ways among different people, and influenced by many factors.

Meanwhile, there have been links found between specific behaviors and various measures of wellbeing. For example, improvements in self-esteem can lead to an immediate change in physiology [12]. Higher self-esteem correlates with higher vagal tone, a measurement of the cardiovascular system. We need to care for ourselves because feeling better about ourselves can directly improve our health.

Furthermore, researchers are increasingly finding that strategies such as mindfulness, self-compassion, resilience and empathy can help people manage their feelings. They have also shown to decrease burnout and improve stress management[13]. These positive traits are among those that contribute to loving oneself.

Why is it important to love yourself? If you don't love yourself, and accept yourself and your feelings, you'll never be able to be fully loved by anyone [14]. Drs. Gay and Kathlyn Hendricks have been psychologists in practice for a combined 90 years. They have seen tens of thousands of patients and students in their trainings and countless viewers on Oprah Winfield's TV shows. They hold this verdict through their considerable experience and many other treating professionals share this view as well. Valuing your partner happens when you value yourself.

Loving yourself includes caring for yourself. Self-care is increasingly found to enable people to accomplish positive things, such as, performing medical care on an ongoing basis for their own chronic conditions to supporting people to perform at their best in their daily activities.

How do you love yourself?

One way is to be grateful you are human. Be grateful for having had a great time with someone at some time. Appreciate the really amazing experiences in your life. Then, contemplate why you are grateful for them and get the deeper reasons.

Another way is to get quiet and go inside yourself, which means sense the inside of your body and tune in to the warmth of your life inside your body. Feel that 98.6 degrees inside your body that comes from your body processing your life within yourself. Connect to that as your source of life and the source of your energy. See in all of this, that there are no good or bad parts of you. There is simply life pulsing inside of you. You might think your body has shortcomings, most everyone does. But take a step further and recognize that your body is working to keep you alive. Appreciate that and love yourself for this.

Realize you get what you believe. Look at your positive beliefs, favorite experiences, most enjoyed people, and the times you felt love in your life. Make a list of them and review it regularly to create and practice a routine of reviewing self-caring thoughts. Counter the many times we heard negative messages about ourselves with positive messages.

Relationship researcher Dr. Gottman says we need five times as many positive messages to counteract negative ones. So tip the balance in our self view towards positive and towards self-love.

Another way is to think of a person, an acquaintance, a celebrity, or someone we don't know personally but know of and consider things we love about them. Then adapt those characteristics into our own life and behave in those ways. When you increase the traits you love, you'll tip your self-view to the loving range.

We can love ourselves with a brief technique to practice daily for a period of time, such as a week [15]:

- Think of someone or something you know you love.
- Feel the love you have for that person or thing.
- Love yourself in exactly the same way. Move the love on to yourself.
- Feel that love.
- Scan your body and sense if there's any place that feels hard to love.
- If you feel a place that seems unloved, give it a moment of loving.
- Just add a drop of love to it.
- Take a breath to add that place to the rest of yourself.

Let go of unloving messages you tell yourself.

Forgive yourself for everything that disappoints you about yourself. You can tackle these last two ways to love yourself on your own, but the path will be easier and faster if you work with a life coach or therapist.

Commitment to loving yourself is a commitment to taking full responsibility for yourself, your life and the results, including the quality of your relationship [16]. Loving yourself is the one thing you can do on your own to improve the quality of your relationship, your wellbeing and the quality of your life. And that can really seem magical.

*"Think of someone or something you know you love.
Feel the love you have for that person or thing.
Now, love yourself exactly the same way."*
~ Gay Hendricks, Ph.D. ~

Amy Carter

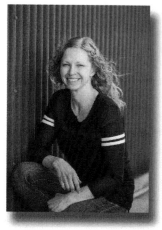

Amy Carter is a certified nutrition coach, personal trainer, and personal growth coach with more than ten years of experience in the health and fitness industry.

A mother of four, triathlete, and foodie who struggled with her own health, she eventually discovered the secrets to balancing her life; restoring her own health, and has recently initiated a program to help others do the same.

"To keep the body in good health is a duty...
otherwise we shall not be able to keep our mind strong and clear."
~ Buddha ~

South Jordan, Utah, USA

Website: www.mybeautifulbalancedlife.com/home-page-offer

Social Media:
- www.facebook.com/behealthymehealthywe/
- www.linkedin.com/in/amy-carter-6ab83686/
- www.medium.com/@amyelizabethcarter

Ready to upgrade your health, and take back your life? Schedule a 30-minute blueprint session with me! https://balancedbodyblueprint.com/go

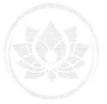

Use The C.U.P. Method To Transform Your Health And Life

Are You Running On Full, Or Empty?

I am an optimist, mother, and nutritious foodie. But life changed in 2018 when I set out to lose the last five pounds by means of extreme endurance training and food restriction. I developed a sudden heart condition that required surgery to repair and restore its normal function. I'd unknowingly hit rock bottom.

Everything I thought I knew about nutrition, exercise, and weight loss came crashing down! I had to start from scratch and understand there is so much more to weight loss, health and wellness than diet and exercise alone. I didn't realize how necessary filling my cup is, and to fill it with the right things, for my health, my family, and a joyful, fulfilling life. And I mean an overflowing, abundant life, not a half-full, relatively happy, mediocre life.

So, I began researching and studying balance. I found the most successful and sustainable habits, in health and in life, are not based on an all-or-nothing approach, but on individual values and goals, desires, investments; like disciplined effort and time, understanding, ability, and necessity.

Are you feeling like you are running on empty? As if you were chasing one rabbit in twenty different directions, trying to do so much, but accomplishing little? I too felt this way, until I learned to create balance by finding strength in imperfections. This was something I had feared and ignored. Now, I needed that strength more than ever.

Wherever you're reaching to find balance, there are three essential principles that must become your new standard, to achieve balance for an upgrade in your health, wealth, relationships, and life. These principles make up the C.U.P. Method, and are applicable to your health, relationships and growth in every reach of your life!

Let's dive into this method, one step at a time.

CONSISTENCY: Knowing When To Do What's Necessary For Success

Hands down, the most dominant choices of everyday life are driven more by consistent and repetitive behavior than by a cost and benefit analysis. This is why even the most desirable goals are often initiated, only to quickly rundown, like a temporary glitch in a fine-tuned motor of habit.

If this is the case, how do we change those habits? Through the development of triggers, anchors, and deliberate discipline we call, consistency.

When we speak of consistency, we don't mean the texture of Jell-O or chocolate pudding. Rather, it means a disciplined practice of the same principles, course, etc. It also means your actions are in harmony among parts of a more complex system. This is where your values, knowledge, and discipline, strengthen one another.

It also means we embrace, not run from, the discomfort of raising our game. To not have a perfect knowledge, but to have faith in your imperfect action. Know our imperfections are required to raise those practices to a level of strength which ultimately brings us to a level of life necessary to sustain those high performance habits.

You cannot sustain the amount of $1 million, without also consistently practicing the habits of a millionaire. Likewise, you cannot sustain a healthy lifestyle without sustainable, consistent practices that create that healthy lifestyle.

If by now you are feeling the need for some introspection and don't know where to start to move forward with consistency in your habits, take heart. You are not alone and you are not without help.

To give you somewhere to start, here are some questions to help you raise the requirement for consistency in your efforts, and begin today to create a real strategy towards your greater goals in your health and life.

- What goals, when done consistently help me to live my highest self and achieve my greatest vision?

- Who needs me to raise myself to these requirements (My true motives)?

- What does my consistent best look like?

- What will I do starting today- right now - to practice consistency and raise the requirement for transformation in my health and life?

UNDERSTANDING: The What and Why We Do

Long before I became a nutrition, fitness, and personal growth coach, I knew being healthy was important, but I didn't really understand why I wanted to be healthy. It wasn't until I gained almost 40 pounds my Freshman year that I realized my whys, and had a better understanding of the reasons for reaching that goal. Being more than 40 pounds overweight, I knew then I no longer wanted to feel too big for my clothes, sluggish, uncomfortable, and unable to think clearly.

One tool I have developed over the last few years to dig deep and figure out what my whys and whats are, is "My Personal PEAK Goal Sheet." It's often the deliberation of how we can do something that gets us into the rut of procrastination and frustration, running around in circles like a hamster running frantically on a wheel to nowhere. When you are willing to put in a little cerebral effort to figuring out the whys and whats, which are often the real results of our dreams and aspirations, the hows then easily fall into place.

PRACTICE: The Strategy, Or HOW, To Achieve Results

We have learned by now it's not enough to know something; knowledge, or understanding, is only potential power towards accomplishing the goals of weight loss, improved health, better relationships, and a more fulfilled life.

I've got a good sense that because you are reading this book, you are already self-motivated and willing to do something to upgrade your health and your life. You are inspired by others who have done the same, and you're willing to do what it takes to change.

But what do you do?

Defining those strategies is the task at hand. For example, one strategy I have incorporated because balance is so important in my personal health is to give my body more time to rest between meals. This works really well for my body to efficiently use the fat-energy system.

Remember, your practice is as unique and individual as you are, you know this is true deep down because you've tried following someone else's "diet plan", someone else's tactics, only to quit or be miserable because they are not your own!

To create sustainable habits, we have to first consider what influences these routines in your own life so you can shift your mindset, your emotions, and change your environment for long-term, successful strategies.

Conclusion

We've almost come full circle; addressing the crucial commitment to consistent, deliberate practice, the understanding of why we are committed to the everyday, important discipline to build strong, sustainable habits.

In order to complete the circle and keep it running smoothly along an occasionally bumpy, smooth, or winding path to the top, you will need to have those routines and systems built upon the foundation of this formula as a fundamental piece to complete the cycle, and give power and purpose to your actions. The routines and systems will reduce distraction, remove limitations, and boost your ability and confidence with each step you successfully perform. After all, you are capable of doing extraordinary things!

You are a remarkable person, and doing that little extra with the C.U.P. Method to fill your cup, improve your health, and increase your impact, there is no limit to the transformation, from the ordinary to the extraordinary, you can experience!

"Everything starts with a thought. Your thoughts become things, and anything that your mind can conceive, you can achieve."
~ Charlamagne tha God ~

Kelli Hirt

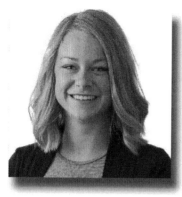

Kelli is a Certified Health Education Specialist (CHES) who values genuine connection with others as a part of her personal and professional life.

She believes community and trust are cultivated through individual conversations which meet people where they are.

This, Kelli believes, is important when implementing successful individual and community interventions in public health areas she is passionate about, including the food system, behavioral, mental, and sexual health.

She is currently pursuing a Master of Public Health degree from the University of Minnesota and has ambitious goals of changing the way America addresses certain health topics related to prevention.

"Be kinder to yourself, then let your kindness flood the world."
~ Pema Chodrön !

Minneapolis, Minnesota, USA

Social Media:
- www.linkedin.com/in/kelli-hirt-ches-9244a1106/

Together, let's create a culture that is more understanding of individuals' health needs. kelli.hirt@gmail.com

The Fear of Facing Judgment: Stigma's Impact on Health

It seems that the most trivial things in life are neither memorable nor traumatizing; my first OB-GYN appointment was an exception.

After nearly seven years of dealing with intense menstrual pain that would often keep me from getting out of bed, I found myself sitting in a sterile hospital waiting room with my mom quietly dwelling on the unfairness of my situation. I was not here by choice; my mom finally convinced me to see an OB-GYN to understand the cause of my menstrual pain. It felt strange that at the age of seventeen I had to confront the realities of reproductive health complications and the self-advocacy that was needed to properly address them.

While the gynecologist was thorough and offered medically-sound remedies to my complications, I was not in the right mindset to either appreciate or absorb the information. As a teenage girl, I was supposed to be, quote-on-quote, "normal," or at least that's what I thought was expected of me. I left the appointment feeling distraught, embarrassed, and defeated. As my mom drove me home, I couldn't help but cry. It felt as though years of shame over my problematic reproductive health and fear to seek help finally boiled over; it was at this moment I knew I needed further help.

This realization did not manifest quickly, however. Years later, this shame reemerged when I sought mental health counseling as a junior in college. Though I felt directionless and wanted professional guidance at this time, I kept down-playing my struggle because, arguably, other people had it worse. I began to realize this monopolization of human pain is only the product of social pressure, exacerbated by stigma, to be "normal."

In this way, my story is not unique; the pursuit of normalcy heightens feelings of shame, fear, and embarrassment in all facets of human culture. This is especially true with topics centered on health and wellness. Nonetheless, I found the more

I built out my support systems for my physical and mental conditions and had conversations surrounding them, I felt less alone and more empowered to help others.

As an emerging health educator, I've witnessed what the impact stigma has in academic, social, and work environments. Stigma can be both outstanding or subtle, but usually debilitating for those who must deal with it. In fact, the Mayo Clinic notes that "discrimination can be a result of stigma, which may manifest itself in people making negative comments about someone's mental illness or avoiding someone because you 'assume they are unstable' when it comes to mental illness [1]". My lived experience qualifies this claim; discrimination and stigma are common issues for people dealing with any condition not well understood by the public.

In the context of public health, real or perceived stigma can reduce the success of preventative health efforts related to, among others, mental and sexual health, substance abuse, and LGBTQ+ individuals. The Mayo Clinic lists a few harmful effects of stigma that are not exclusive to any one condition but include reluctance to seek treatment, inability to find work opportunities, inadequacy of health insurance coverage, and a misunderstanding from family, friends, or coworkers [2].

The same goes for our healthcare system; a systematic literature review reveals stigma might hinder healthcare processes in medical facilities, noting that its manifestations are widely documented. Because of the discrimination associated with stigma, patients with abnormal health conditions are more likely to be denied services, face purposely longer wait times, and endure physical or verbal abuse. As such, those with stigmatized conditions have difficulty maintaining a healthy quality of life (QOL) [3].

Barriers to healthcare result in poorer well-being. The Centers for Disease Control and Prevention show that well-being contributes to multiple outcomes related to QOL, including social connectedness, productivity, and longevity [4]. The problems which stigma creates for the country as a whole are greater than meets the eye. When social connectedness is compromised, so it our health. More isolation from stigma could mean more chronic disease, driving up healthcare costs, reducing individual and community productivity, and overall well-being.

Reducing stigma is not an easy task but it is vital to improve the population's well-being and further increase access to comprehensive services. There is no universal answer to reducing stigma but we can collectively start somewhere.

Nelson Mandela said it best: "Education is the most powerful weapon which you can use to change the world."

Fundamentally, education develops empowered people who advocate for better health for themselves and others through knowledge and experience. Empowered people are productive people. Empowered people have the ability to effect positive, personal, and community change; thereby igniting a cultural shift. Basic education, formal or informal, has the potential to motivate people to take care of, and prioritize, their health so they can have the option to live as their healthiest self without fear of discrimination. Additionally, it has the power to build allies who, when it comes to stigma, can help break down societal beliefs surrounding health conditions we are so hesitant to discuss.

As individuals, you and I can begin to break down these barriers in several ways.

First, we can strive to be more honest and compassionate with ourselves, even under the pressure stigma creates. Embracing vulnerability while facing my fears of rejection and embarrassment drove my passion for identifying and reducing stigma to pave the way for others to do the same.

Second, we can use this compassion to become better allies by cultivating a greater understanding of how stigma presents itself and affects our ability to seek needed treatment.

Third, as allies, we can begin to initiate open conversations with each other to normalize sensitive health related conditions, leading to a cultural shift in beliefs.

For those of us who are dealing with the effects of stigma, it is important to identify a supportive network to be present throughout the healing process. It is crucial for these networks to understand both the facts of our unique situations and the type of care we need.

For people who are support systems: Being there to encourage and actively listen without judgment to the people who are dealing with stigma can be enough for them to seek professional treatment needed. Remember, there is no timeline for right or wrong when it comes to taking charge of your health. For me, it took five years after my seemingly horrifying OB-GYN appointment to continue learning more about my conditions and actively work at correcting them.

Overcoming stigma is a daunting task, but it can be achieved. Knowing yourself at both your weakest and strongest point can only happen when you choose to make your health a priority. If I had known ten years ago what I know now, I would have encouraged myself to break the social barriers to achieve a better understanding of my health conditions sooner. I would tell myself, like I am telling you now, that you are worth more than the debilitating effects of stigma. You are worth starting your journey to a better you, and you don't have to do it alone.

Vivianne Romang

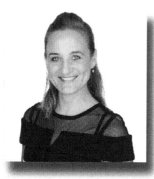

Vivianne works with clients in Switzerland and Internationally to help them master their emotions and connect with themselves in a healthier way so that they may enjoy a balanced and fulfilling experience of life.

In addition to her Emotional Mastery Training Programs, she also teaches her own form of dynamic Yoga.

Using the tools of Yoga, meditation, pranayama and intensive self-study, Vivianne turned her life from a seemingly endless emotional roller-coaster mired by stress in the workplace, PTSD from childhood abuse, and chronic illness, to a life that inspires and drives me forward.

These tools naturally developed over the years into the Yoga@Home and Emotional Mastery@Home coaching programs that she now teaches both online and in person.

"If your mind carries a heavy burden of past,
you will experience more of the same.
The past perpetuates itself through lack of presence.
The quality of your consciousness at this moment is what shapes the future."
~ Eckhart Tolle ~

Savigny, Vaud, Switzerland

Website: www.beyondillusions.ch/

Social Media:
- www.facebook.com/vivianneromangyoga
- www.instagram.com/vivianne.romang/
- www.linkedin.com/in/vivianneteachingandlearning/

Contact Vivianne today for a free consultation to find out if Emotional Mastery Training is for you vivianne@beyondillusions.ch

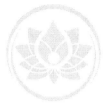

The Six Pillars of Stress Management for Immune Support

Most of us who have arrived at the point where we turn to natural and organic forms of healing, are doing so after having exhausted all other possibilities. We have taken our prescribed medication, and visited countless doctors without experiencing long-lasting and integrative wellbeing.

Medicine has made amazing advances such as 3-D printed prosthetics, robotic surgery, and precision medicine; a personalised medicine that attacks tumours based on the patient's specific genes and proteins. However, when it comes to health, we are still focussed much more on treating the symptoms of illness rather than prevention, promoting wellness or dealing with the root causes.

We now know that chronic stress is one of the biggest threats to immune function, the immune system being our actual defence system for the body to ward off disease. A research team led by Carnegie Mellon University's, Sheldon Cohen, found that the effects of psychological stress on the body's ability to regulate inflammation can promote the development and progression of disease [1].

Therefore, it is essential to decrease and limit chronic stress in our lives in order to support our body's natural ability to heal.

People suffer from chronic stress in various different ways:

- Constant work overload
- Effects of a childhood trauma
- Post-Traumatic-Stress-Disorder (PTSD)
- Suffering a traumatic injury that leads to physical inability
- Being a prisoner of war
- A victim of abuse
- etc.

However, if you have ever experienced chronic stress, I think you will agree it is not always easy or possible to undo the stressor, let alone recognize you are even suffering from this chronic condition.

Apart from that, we all react differently to different stressors. What causes stress for one person may actually be a motivator for another. It is therefore of greater interest and importance that we focus on how to deal with stress rather than on making stress the culprit. We must apply our innate human capacity of consciousness to deal better with stress.

In order to help with this task, I have highlighted six pillars of stress management to support our health; we can view these as beneficial habits to train.

The six pillars of stress-management for immune support:

1. Awareness
2. Beliefs & Interpretation
3. Reasoning
4. Thoughts
5. Breath & Somatic Awareness
6. Emotions

These habits are interlinked, each one affects or influences the other. So, when one is not functioning properly, the others will suffer too. But, when one is functioning properly, it will positively impact the others.

1. Awareness

One of the ways in which chronic stress manages to pervade our lives is due to the fact that we are greatly unaware. Unaware of our emotions, unaware of our thoughts, unaware of our physiological responses, unaware of how our body even 'feels'.

Without awareness, nothing changes. We will simply keep reacting on auto-pilot, whether it is beneficial to our health or not. Awareness is the first and vital step which will allow us to recognize how we may have added to our own illness; whether through diet, lack of exercise, or in the case of our inner world, emotions, thoughts and beliefs.

Practical Tip

Set aside one precise point each day (you can set an alarm on your phone if it helps) at which you ask yourself:

- "How do I feel?"
- "How does this (whatever is going on) affect me?"
- "How do I feel about myself?"
- "How do I feel about life?"
- "What is going on inside me?"

This will give you a moment to notice if there are things that need to be changed in order for you to feel better. It will also help you feel less attached to situations or feelings of distress. Awareness itself already loosened their grip.

2. Beliefs & Interpretation

Consciousness allows us to interpret our experiences. These interpretations can be beneficial, or non-beneficial, to our health and wellbeing. They can cause stress or offer relief. It is up to us as to how we choose to interpret our experiences. Changing interpretation can change everything!

Practical Tip

When we are ill or not feeling well, we tend to view our body, or ourselves, as 'the enemy', the foreign vessel that is taking all our energy. Instead of viewing illness or our body as the enemy, we could take feeling unwell as the body sending us a message.

"My body is my friend. My body is sending me a message – what is it telling me?"

You are neglecting your own needs. Change how you treat yourself. Change how you speak to yourself. Don't fight your body. Listen to how you are feeling. Love yourself. Have patience with yourself. Be kind, not only to others but above all, be kind to yourself.

Or, you may be someone who interprets your experience through the lens of your own identity, your beliefs about yourself. For example, if you feel like circumstances happen to you and which you have no control over, you play the victim role. You will feel weak and ill, you will expect to keep experiencing this. This too, as with your interpretations, can be turned inside out, questioned and finally challenged. Choose the beliefs that support growth and drop those that keep you stuck.

This is your body speaking. From now on, thank your body for the message. From now on, do not hear – but listen!

3. Reasoning

This relates closely with beliefs & interpretation. Instead of being angry at the fact you may not experience overnight healing, apply reason. Reason will tell you that you have exposed yourself to years of stress, perhaps even decades of emotional turmoil, an incessant roller-coaster of thoughts and emotions. It goes to reason therefore, that it may take some time to reset your body from illness to optimum health.

Practical Tip

Apply the first point, awareness, to notice when you are feeling improvement. Notice even the small steps. Notice these especially when you are feeling unwell, and remind yourself to be patient. Remind yourself how long you lived unaware, battering your body. Remind yourself that years of ill treatment will take time to undo.

4. Thoughts

Ah yes, thoughts! Thoughts are completely linked with reasoning and awareness. However, we can have so many thoughts that we are unaware of. For optimum health, we are interested in shaping our thoughts more consciously. It is as simple as this: some thoughts make us feel good and some thoughts make us feel bad. Choosing the thoughts that make us feel good can transform a moment of stress into a neutral experience, or even a motivator.

Practical Tip

Dedicate to paying more attention to your thoughts. When you don't feel good, ask yourself "what thoughts drive this feeling?"

Use your daily moments of awareness to then begin to question your thoughts and their validity. Instead of believing your negative thought, ask "how can I change this thought to help me feel better?" Sometimes all it takes is flipping a thought and looking at it from a different angle to release its negative hold on you.

5. Breath / Somatic Awareness

In yoga, breath regulation is one of the primary paths to greater awareness, presence, and mental and physical health. Not only does each breathing exercise have its own specific therapeutic effects on our physiology, but breath regulation in general helps us adjust our thoughts, our emotions, and tensions in the body.

You may wish to take some pranayama classes in which you learn specific breathing exercises, these would be a huge boost to your health!

Practical Tip

Next time you notice yourself feeling unpleasant in some way – upset, angry, anxious, fearful, overwhelmed – notice how your breath changes. Noticing the changes in your breath will already bring some calm. See if you can breathe more deeply, more slowly. Inhale deeply, count your inhale, and then exhale as slowly as you can. Counting your exhale, see if you can lengthen it beyond the count of your inhale. Can you get to two extra counts? Three? Or can you practice this often enough to double your exhale in ratio to your inhale?

As you notice your breath, notice your posture. Notice your shoulders and your neck. Notice your face. Notice your forehead. Notice your jaw. Where do you hold tension? How does this tension serve you? Does it serve you? Keep up with the breathing and allow yourself to let the tension go.

6. Emotions

Emotions…ooooh, yes, emotions! Some of us are completely overwhelmed by our emotions whilst others are seemingly immune to them. Either way, if we can relate to one of these ways of 'dealing with' emotions, then we are in fact unaware of our emotions and not dealing with them at all. Once again, all our habits are linked.

Emotions are this huge melting pot, fed and influenced by our awareness, or lack thereof; our thoughts, our beliefs, our interpretations… everything can negatively impact our emotions, if we allow it to! However, emotions only carry the weight that we allow them to. Emotions can be fleeting and pass through us like air. Or they can be stored inside and grow like a cancer. This final element is probably one of the most important to deal with, and it is the one that is completely dependent on all the others.

When we become more conscious of all the aforementioned habits, we will automatically become more aware of our emotions and less attached to them. We will give them less permission to control our health both mental and physical.

We will be freer - We will be more connected to our true nature.

Kelly Brickel

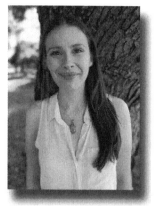

Kelly Brickel is a Certified Reiki Master Teacher, Master Practitioner of NLP and MER®, and Certified Teacher of Psychic and Mediumship development through Lisa Williams' International School of Spiritual Development (LWISSD).

She works as a Reiki Healer, Psychic-Medium, Numerologist, Mentor, and Spiritual Coach.

Kelly's passions are working with Spirit and healing energy.

She loves teaching and helping others find the beauty and strength of their gifts, whether it be becoming a reader, healer, or more intuitive with their own lives.

"A person's health isn't generally a reflection of genes, but how their environment is influencing them. Genes are the direct cause of less than 1% of diseases: 99% is how we respond to the world."
~ Dr. Bruce Lipton ~

Lake Forest, California, USA

Website: www.EnergeticSessions.com

Social Media:
- www.facebook.com/energeticsessions
- www.instagram.com/kellybrickel/
- www.linkedin.com/in/kellybrickel/

To schedule a reading, healing, or contact Kelly visit: www.energeticsessions.com

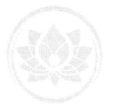

Healing with Reiki

What is Reiki?

Reiki is in definition, a complementary energetic healing modality. It has a rich background with origins from Japan, China, Tibet, and other asian regions dating back thousands of years. In the early 1900's there was a resurgence of Reiki in Japan, which largely is where people connect to and typically identify with what they know of Reiki's roots.

This energy healing style has grown into a well known therapy tool for aiding in relaxation, rejuvenation, and holistic connection. Reiki itself can include hands-on healing or no physical contact within a session. Although Reiki loosely translates to "Universal Life Force Energy" in english, it is formed from Japanese Kanji from the words Rei and Ki and actually has a more open-ended meaning that isn't limited to one translation.

Kanji is one part of the Japanse writing system where characters are formed into picture symbols rather than holding a specific definition. Two Kanji symbols can be combined to form a compound meaning or idea. Various translations help shape the ideas of Reiki and can give it justice with deeper clarity.

When the Japanese characters of Rei and Ki come together it symbolizes bridging heaven and earth. Rei symbolizes the collecting of the heavens and Ki, vital life force energy; bringing purpose through the act of bridging the two for harmonious function.

Above guiding below, the Universe enlightening the earth as it receives, the Divine or the mystery igniting, sparking life force. There are many interpretations.

Whether from being a receiver or a practitioner of Reiki, when one learns about this energy and allows Reiki to flow through their body, they will grow to know that it comes from a place of the most positive intentions.

History of Reiki

The most common form of Reiki typically found is influenced from traditional Usui Reiki. Many Practitioners in Japan and the United States practice this style which was introduced by a man named Mikao Usui.

Since originating in Japan during the early 1920's, this form of Reiki (Usui) has been practiced and passed down from generations of a lineage of teachers.

Mikao Usui had a long background in studying Philosophy, Religion, and History. He was a lover of a diverse range of studies. His upper class upbringing gave him opportunities to an extensive and ongoing education; which his personality relished in. Mikao developed his interest in Metaphysics and Healing Arts as side passion for many years before developing Usui Reiki. In fact, he was 57 years old at the time of its inception.

During a profound turn in his personal spiritual development and meditations, Mikao was compelled to share his revelations with others so they could equally benefit. With such, he developed a new style of an ancient art. In 1922, soon after his epiphany and success with utilizing these techniques, Usui developed an institute which included a school and clinic where he taught practitioners and healed incoming patients. His incentive for building the institute was for everyday people to receive the healing benefits of Reiki, and believed that it should not be an exclusive treatment to the educated or privileged. His enlightenment gave him clarity to pursue this conviction.

In 1923, Tokyo experienced a devastating earthquake in the Kanto district, close to where Usui's clinic was located. Usui and his practitioners aided and helped locals heal and recover from the aftermath. Within 3 years, by 1925, Usui's training and clinic institute was gaining so many patients and students, they expanded to a new and larger location.

Many people had heard and sought training with Reiki from Usui's school and his reputation continued to grow. 45 years later, Reiki spread to the United States largely from Hawaii and California. By the 1970's, through personal experiences and word of mouth, it began to root and flourish in the West. Since that time, many styles and variations have formed from traditional Usui Reiki, just like Usui sprouted from other Reiki traditions.

Mikao Usui's impact with Reiki is undeniable and is responsible for many of the current foundations and traditions still found in Japan, and particularly, the United States.

How Does Reiki Work?

Let's get into it. The practitioner facilitating the session begins by running Reiki through his or her body, then working with the client's body/energy field to help alleviate highlighted concerns. This can be done in a professional setting using a massage table or with a chair where the patient remains fully clothed during the session.

The practitioner, with permission of the client, lays their hands gently upon, or above the client's body sensing information coming from areas of the physical/ energetic body. Depending on an individual practitioner's training, they may connect to their client's energy in different ways.

During Reiki, practitioners mix their Ki with universal energy to generate and ground healing states stemming from the synergy of an energy that is greater than one's individual self. For many people, this synergy which does not have a concrete definition and is likened to thoughts of a collective source of intelligence, the universe, a higher power such as a belief in God, sacred or divine origin, or a connective force that is present within all beings. When we are connected to this force, our energy receives from a source of energy collective.

Individuals who experience Reiki describe sessions as soothing and revitalizing in more ways than just physical. The energy received helps to balance emotional, mental, and spiritual areas of a person's makeup.

Reiki helps returning/resetting ourselves to a deeper state of harmony than it was prior. It is the nature of our state of being to have ups and downs; everyone of us has excessive flow or depletions of energy in our bodies. Alternative therapies such as Acupuncture and Acupressure similarly acknowledge this belief. Blockages surface from energetic inconsistencies and are thought to emerge from our environment, subconscious/conscious beliefs, and how we process them. The range of how our energy moves throughout our body is in connection to our fears, personal or influenced belief systems, memories, repetitive or flowing thoughts, expressed or suppressed emotions; the patterns of our life shape our energy.

We all have energy patterns. When energy is healthy, it feels even, flowing, there is a gentle, soft movement, a harmonious distribution. Blockages in the body are related to excessive or depleted flow. When blockages are present, energy can feel spiky, heavy or staticy. Think of an Olympic athlete over-exerting themselves in bursts. It's an interesting display, a surge of energy, but the body cannot sustain itself on that output 24/7. Now, think of a chronically inactive person, their vitality will be weak from such a state, their muscle memory of performing certain tasks will atrophy over time.

Overactive and underactive areas point to unhealthy processes within the body; blocked flow of Ki/Chi. The goal of Reiki is to share energy greater than one's self to exponentially increase flow within the body/energetic field. This way the natural healing properties within ourselves can be reinvigorated and harmonized.

Common experiences during a Reiki session are:

- Feeling a rush of heat, cold, or tingling within one's body
- Feeling a current or movement within the one's body
- Feeling a soothing, calming energy, that reduces tension and heaviness
- Feelings of mental ease or emotional positivity

Frequent results shared after several treatments:

- Boosted energy levels
- Deep relaxation that lasts several days or longer
- Feeling more supported in life
- Mental clarity and awareness
- Being more proactive
- Experiencing life in a positive, lighter, and healthier perspective

Reiki can help adults, children, and animals in coping with stress in everyday life and other circumstances. Hospitals, clinics, and hospices are using Reiki increasingly as a Complementary Therapy and treatment within Alternative and Allopathic Medicine.

Tips to Find a Reiki Practitioner

It is highly recommended that you research and find recommendations for a Reiki practitioner if you are seeking a session. Every practitioner leans to specialties as different parts of the body function with different subtleties.

If you are not seeking a generalized session, identify the reason why you are having Reiki to help find the right kind of practitioner. Reiki practitioners that have been working routinely for 2-3 years or more with multiple recommendations are a great way to find a quality session.

Most individuals that have been working this long will be Reiki Masters. Another important mention is to not choose someone based on their Reiki Master title. An overzealous practitioner can receive their Master training in mere months. Experience, time, and recommendations are key to a wonderful experience.

Reiki Maintenance

If you find a Reiki session benefits you, the typical follow-up is every 6 months to a year. For a specified or chronic issue, the session can be once a week, month, or every other month.

Reiki focuses on different processes with one's overall body. A standard Reiki session is a general overview and healing, supplemented by feedback from the practitioner with details of your physical and energetic body.

More specified sessions consist of the practitioner working with an emphasis on the physical body or the other "subtle bodies."

An example with physical emphasis being an injury, recent surgery, or muscle pain. For the mental body, focals point being the head region, issues of headaches, depression, or cycling thoughts/ memories.

Within the emotional body, an example of emphasis would be to help with processing emotions and the changing of relationships.

A spiritually based session would focus on finding clarity in direction in life as well as working with the upper regions of a person's energy that contribute to visions, epiphanies and awareness.

Reiki is one branch of a great tree, however energetic healing attracts your interest, know there are quality options out there to engage in with your energetic healing experiences.

Many practitioners such as myself, have a great heart in this work and are excited to play their part in sharing the wonders of Reiki.

Vivian Jalique

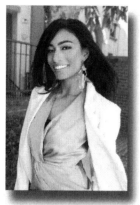

Vivian Jalique is holistic wellness and spirituality coach based out of Union City, California.

As a single mother, she wishes to inspire her daughter to go after her dreams no matter how hard the road may be.

She began her journey as a meditation guide and Reiki Practitioner in 2012. Vivian is also a certified massage therapist and health educator since March 2014.

She has been developing her brand, based off this chapter title "The Love Manual", which is focused, but not limited to, women's holistic and spiritual health.

Her mission in life is to empower women in understanding the ways of healing their heart, body, mind and soul through self love practices.

"Love is happy when it is able to give something.
The ego is happy when it is able to take something."
~ Osho ~

Union City, California, USA

Website: www.mylovemanual.com

Social Media:
- www.instagram.com/mylovemanual
- www.facebook.com/mylovemanual

Jumpstart your journey towards authentic self love. www.mylovemanual.com

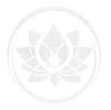

My Love Manual

What is self love, and how do you love yourself? How do you know when you love yourself enough while making it an authentic experience? Is it vain to love oneself?

These are a few of the questions I would ask myself from time to time. I have come to discover that the answers are simple, but your ego will be challenged and torn apart in so many ways.

When I first began my journey on the path of self love three years ago, I really meditated on these thoughts. I began to seek guidance through self love videos, people, and multiple books. Through my observations of what I was absorbing, as well as, observing myself through retaining these methods, I learned there isn't one way of loving yourself. It is not something you do just once, or even a few times, and become completely sound. No, it is a journey that will break you down and make you face your deepest truths, and every time you say yes to self love, it empowers you more and more. Self love is never vain, so long as you are reaching from your heart space and not the ego. The question is, can you identify your ego?

Identifying The Negative Ego Influences

What is The Ego?

The ego is not our true selves but the mask we wear in life which we use to navigate through our earth bound society. It is manifested through an illusion of self. We have attained through our experiences, traumas, and the relationships that created a major impact in our life, shaping us into who we "are". Often times, we mistake our ego for our true selves.

In my belief, we cannot be 100% free of our ego until we leave this human body. The ego's main objective is to protect you at any means necessary, even if it means making you feel insecure and lacking self love in order to keep you from your pain. However; you must love yourself through this pain, as love will help you see the true message in your journey. It is important that we become aware of our influences and what it does to our ego.

Influences

When we become aware of our influences, it is easier to change your influences to more positive ones. You will find your ego's voice is silenced through more positive influences.

I do this practice with myself where once a month where I take a moment to observe with a pen and paper, voice recording, or a digital platform. I start by observing what, where, and who is a daily part of my life in the month and how that affects my wellbeing. In my listing, if I find something or someone weighs my energy down, I let it go for good, or I allow myself space if I wish to return to it when a positive energy shift has happened. This practice keeps me on my toes and keeps me mindful. How does your influences affect you?

Here is an example:
Of course; when you are surrounded by people who gossip and degrade others, you will begin to feel drained. Perhaps you may begin justifying yourself to gossip about others too. However, what good does that do for you and those involved? Imagine now that you are surrounded with people who empower one another and praise each other on one another's talents and achievements. Imagine these people sharing knowledge, as well as offering guidance to help balance one another out. [This is an example is based on the Master Mind which you can find more information about through the book " The Law of Success" by Napoleon Hill.] How do you think that positive influence can change your life?

Reflection Questions
- What people influence your life? Is it positive or negative? What type of people do you want to influence your life and why?
- What environments are influencing your life, such as your home, work space, and recreational spaces? Is it positive or negative? What type of environment do you want to influence your life and why?
- What thoughts influence your life? Consider that this may require you to meditate to reveal these thoughts? What are the negative thoughts that influence you? What positive thoughts can you use to replace those thoughts?

I have a free exercise to help you map out you mental influences and a practice to rewire and replace your negative thought. Please see my website for further information.

Heal and Love Your Heart -Affirmations

What are affirmations?

Affirmations are the practice of positive thinking and self validation aimed towards confidence of the self, how ever it is wished to be translated. You can write down your own affirmations or follow along with those you feel aligned with. Over time you will find your mindset shifting into a success and self love based mindset.

Writing affirmations is simple. All you need to do is begin with an "I" statement, speak in the present tense, and communicate your statements as clearly as possible so you're brain doesn't seek to misconstrue the message.

Self Love, The Affirmation

- I open and ready to receive these truths.
- I am capable of self love
- I am worthy of unconditional self love.
- Every morning, I wake up and realize that I am a lovable person.
- I love so many things about myself, and I am so happy to be me.
- I am confident in myself, and I always speak my truth with compassion and respect.
- I respect and am compassionate to myself
- Loving myself authentically is so essential to myself growth
- I say yes to myself, because I am responsible for my own happiness
- I take power in that truth and I know that I am the creator of my reality
- Loving myself makes me feel so good
- Loving myself allows me to be fully present with loving others
- I am worth of love
- I am consciously making an effort to love myself every day
- I promise that I will do my best today.

Reflection Questions
- Did you feel best when you spoke the affirmations out loud or in the solitude of your mind?
- Did any feelings come up for you before, during, and after you began affirming yourself?
- Do this consistently for a week. Do you feel any shifts in your mindset?

Heal and Love Your Body - Self Love Chai

The Benefits of Herbs in Your Self Love Practice

Herbal Medicine is a great way to heal your body. There are so many different herbs which are attuned spiritually and physically to the body.

About Self Love Chai

I truly feel that the romance of these two herbs creates a kundalini healing energy within your body which brings peace, bliss, it heals the physical body, heightens the sexual/ creative god bearing energies we all have within us, and so much more. I hope this Chia inspires more self love in you as it has with me. Please feel inspired to add to the blend and share amongst your friends and loved ones.

Self Love Chai Recipe

When I make my tea, I don't really measure it, my apologies. Although, I usually put half the amount of each tea per serving. Thanks for understanding!

Ingredients:
- Damiana loose leaf tea
- Rose bud tea
- (optional) local clover honey or any other preferred sweetener
- (optional) CBD for extra healing benefits
- Almond Milk or substitute
- H2O

Instructions:
1. Boil your water (depending on how many serving you wish to make, put 1-5 cups of water) at medium temp, once it starts to a soft boil, put it on low. You don't want the water too hot boil, it will burn the tea!
2. You don't want the water too hot boil, it will burn the tea!
3. Using a metal or cloth tea bag put in half a measure of Rose Bud tea and half a measure of Damiana tea. Let it steep for fifteen minutes.
4. Once it is steeped, take the tea bag out and put a quarter amount in comparable size to tea.
5. Pour in your cups and add a drop of cbd (optional) and honey to taste (optional)
6. Enjoy the cozy, relaxing, and euphoric influence of the tea!

Reflection Questions:
- Were you able to remain present in this practice? If not, what can you do to prepare in your environment before this practice that will help you stay present?
- What feelings did you notice in your body when drinking Chai?
- Would you like to make changes or have suggestions? If you'd like to share, visit my page and let us know. Thank you in advance!

A Moment of Gratitude

I want you to know that you, as an individual, are vitally important to the universe. You are unique in every way and you have so much within yourself just waiting for your permission to shine through.

No one else can give you that permission but yourself. Validate yourself a powerful force of nature, and use it with the best intentions.

Thank you so much for taking the time to read this chapter. Many blessings to you and yours!

"What drains your spirit drains your body.
What fuels your spirit fuels your body."
~ Carolyn Myss ~

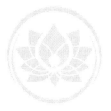

Cited References

Misa Tsuyoshi (pages 6 - 11):
1. https://jenniferdubowsky.com/mayo-clinic-new-research-shows-qigong-can-relieve-chronic-pain/
2. https://www.prweb.com/releases/2010/09/prweb4477844.htm
3. https://www.springforestqigong.com/what-is-qigong
4. https://www.springforestqigong.com/qigong-medical-doctor-testimonials
5. https://www.springforestqigong.com/medical-studies

Kim Farmer (pages 12 - 17):
1. National Alliance On Mental Illness (2019, July 20). Mental Health By the Numbers. Retrieved from http://nami.org

Marquita h Catallo-Madruga (pages 24 - 27):
1. A systematic review of evidence for the added benefits to health of exposure to natural environments D.E. Bowler, LM Buyung-Ali, ™ Knight, AS Pullin. BMC Public Health 10:456 (2010)
2. Article by Terry Hartig from the Lancet in 2018 reviewing a four year longitudinal study by R. Mitchell and F. Popham showed that people in England that had better access to Green Space in the day to day lives had less incidence of cardiovascular disease and Psychological disorders.
3. Selling sickness: the pharmaceutical industry and disease mongering.Ray Moynihan, journalist,a Iona Heath, general practitioner,b and David Henry, professor of clinical pharmacologyc BMJ. 2002 Apr 13; 324(7342): 886–891.

Luanne Nelson (pages 28 - 33):
1. https://ghr.nlm.nih.gov/primer/traits/longevity

Reina Rose (pages 40 - 45):
1. The Wall Street Journal: When Stress at Work Creates Drama at Home https://www.wsj.com/articles/when-stress-at-work-creates-drama-at-

home-11563183015

2. Forbes.com: New Study Shows Correlation Between Employee Engagement And The Long-Lost Lunch Break https://www.forbes.com/sites/alankohll/2018/05/29/new-study-shows-correlation-between-employee-engagement-and-the-long-lost-lunch-break/#77444de94efc

Archana Amlapure (pages 56 - 63):

1. https://www.ncbi.nlm.nih.gov/pubmed/30485713,
2. https://www.ncbi.nlm.nih.gov/pubmed/27702643
3. https://www.who.int/whr/2001/media_centre/press_release/en

Dr. Karen Stillman (pages 70 - 75):

1,4,6,7,8,9. Proctor, Bob, and Mary Morrissey. "Into Your Genius." Training Materials. ©2017

2,3,5,10. Morrissey, Mary. "DreamBuilder® Course." Live DreamBuilder Coach Training, 10 Mar. 2018, Los Angeles, California. Life Mastery Institute.

11. Schucman, Helen. A Course in Miracles: Text, Workbook for Students, Manual for Teachers. IXIA PRESS, 2019.

Aprilani McIlwraith (pages 88 - 93):

1, 3, 6, . Waldinger, R. (2015, November). Robert Waldinger on what makes a good life (Video file). Retrieved from https://www.ted.com/talks/robert_waldinger_what_makes_a_good_life_lessons_from_the_longest_study_on_happiness

2. Holt-Lunstad J, Smith TB, Layton JB. (2010). Social Relationships and Mortality Risk: A Meta-analytic Review. PLoS Med 7(7): e1000316. https://doi.org/10.1371/journal.pmed.1000316

4. Proulx CM, Snyder-Rivas LA. 2013 Apr. The longitudinal associations between marital happiness, problems, and self-rated health. J Fam Psychol. 27(2):194-202. doi: 10.1037/a0031877.

5, 7, . Whisman, M. A., Gilmour, A. L., & Salinger, J. M. (2018). Marital satisfaction and mortality in the United States adult population. Health Psychology, 37(11), 1041-1044.
http://dx.doi.org/10.1037/hea0000677

8. Karimi, R. 2019. The protective factors of marital stability in long-term marriage globally: a systematic review. Epidemiology and Health, e2019023. DOI: https://doi.org/10.4178/epih.e2019023 [Accepted] Published online June 15, 2019. https://www.e-epih.org/journal/view.php?number=1038

9. Gottman, PhD, John D., (December, 2012), Chapter 7: The Four Keys to Improving Your Marriage. Why Marriages Succeed Or Fail: And How You Can Make Yours Last, pp. 175-200. New York, Simon & Schuster.
10. Davoodvandi, M., Navabi Nejad, S., and Farzad, V. 2018 Apr. Examining the Effectiveness of Gottman Couple Therapy on Improving Marital Adjustment and Couples' Intimacy. Iran J Psychiatry. 13(2): 135–141.

11, 14 . Hendricks, PhD, G., Hendricks, PhD, Kathlyn. (January, 1992). Conscious Loving: The Journey To Co-Commitment. New York, Bantam Books.

12. Martens, A., Greenberg, A., & Allen, J.J.B. (2008). Self-esteem and autonomic physiology: Parallels between self-esteem and vagal tone as buffers of threat. Personality and Social Psychology Review, 12, 370-389.

13. Lapa TA, Madeira FM, Viana JS, Pinto-Gouveia J. 2017 Feb. Burnout syndrome and wellbeing in anesthesiologists: the importance of emotion regulation strategies. Minerva Anestesiol. 83(2):191-199. doi: 10.23736/S0375-9393.16.11379-3.

15, 16. Hendricks, PhD, G., (March,1982). Learning to Love Yourself. New York, Atria Books.

Kelli Hirt (pages 100 - 103):
1, 2, . Mayo Clinic. (2017). Mental health: overcoming the stigma of mental illness. Retrieved from: https://www.mayoclinic.org/diseases-conditions/mental-illness/in-depth/mental-health/art-20046477

3. Nyblade, L., Stockton, M., Giger, K., et. Al. (2019). Stigma in health facilities: why it matters and how we can change it. Retrieved from: https://bmcmedicine.biomedcentral.com/articles/10.1186/s12916-019-1256-2

4. Centers for Disease Control and Prevention. (2018). Health Related Quality of Life (HRQOL): Well-Being Concepts. Retrieved from https://www.cdc.gov/hrqol/wellbeing.htm

Vivianne Romang (pages 104 - 109):
1. https://www.cmu.edu/homepage/health/2012/spring/stress-on-disease.shtml

Vivianne Jalique (pages 116 - 121):
1. https://transformationacademy.com/about-us/

"What we don't need in the midst of struggle is shame for being human."
~ Brene Brown ~

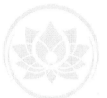

Services Recommended by
The Wellness Fair

Your own personal story will help many people. Do you want to publish it in a book? If you're answer is yes, contact our publisher. They'll make it fast, easy, and affordable for you to get your story out of your head and into print!

Are you an accredited wellness professional?

Then you definitely need to publish a book. Think of the first six letters in the word authority? *USA Today* says 84% of people in the world want to write a book but far less than 1% actually do. Because of that, published authors are:

- Instant experts
- Instant authority figures
- Most trusted source of information
- Increased credibility
- Increased visibility
- ... and much, MUCH, more!

Imagine what that global perception will do for your business!

Authorpreneur Academy will not only make the writing and publishing process fun, quick, and easy, they'll train you on how to leverage your book to build your business before you even write one word!

Not a writer? Most entrepreneurs aren't! They offer a done-for-you service where you show up to just 7 phone calls and they take care of the rest, plus provide free training!

Because they don't work with just anyone, you first need to apply and be interviewed.

Start your book journey by applying today:
https://authorpreneur.academy/apply

"Keep taking time for yourself until you're you again."
~ *Lalah Delia* ~

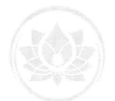

Next Steps

There are many ways you can get involved with our community:

1. *Attend events* as a wellness enthusiasts

2. Consume our *wisdom sharing* materials

3. Be a *vendor* at a local trade fair nearest you

4. Once a vendor, you're able to be a *speaker*

5. Become a *co-author* in the next volume of this book series

6. Contribute to our *guest blog*

7. Contribute to our *quarterly magazine*

8. Be a *guest on our podcast*

9. *Volunteer* to make the events possible

10. *Sponsor* to help our community grow

11. *Get a license* to host events in your area

By partnering with us, you can leverage our community for an entire career; we'll train you how.

Does this seem like something you would be interested in?

Go to **www.TheWellnessFair.org** to join us today!

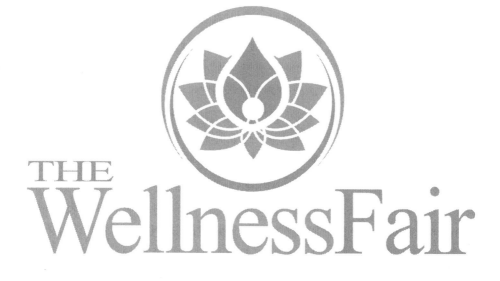

www.TheWellnessFair.org/2019Book

Made in the
USA
Columbia, SC

81938904R00083